Low Carb Diet

The Healthy Way to Lose Weight

Dr. Luis Mispireta

Published in the United States of America

ISBN 979-8-89395-685-6 (SC)
ISBN 979-8-89395-936-9 (Ebook)

Library of Congress Control Number: 2024921996

Mispireta Family Foundation
222 West 6th Street
Suite 400, San Pedro, CA, 90731
www.stellarliterary.com

Order Information and Rights Permission:

Quantity sales. Special discounts might be available on quantity purchases by corporations, associations, and others. For details, contact the publisher at the address above.

For Book Rights Adaptation and other Rights Permission.
Call us at toll-free 1-888-945-8513 or send us an email at admin@stellarliterary.com.

Contents

LOW CARB DIET, THE HEALTHY WAY TO LOSE WEIGHT

Why do we need to diet?

Before discussing diets and weight loss, we must understand why a diet is needed.

During World War II in the US, the rejection of volunteers for the Armed Forces was higher than expected; the cause was that they were underweight. The conclusion was that they were malnourished. The military forces and the government tried to remedy this condition. Several fronts were used for this effort: propaganda, providing sustenance at schools, and recommendations made for ideal meals. It worked very well. The population gained weight; the only problem was gained too much.

Also, since the end of WWII, during the last eighty years, there has been an increase in chronic illnesses such as type 2 diabetes and complications from it, like ischemic cardiac disease and renal failure. The medical profession recognized this and associated it with an average weight gain.

The medical profession and the government adopted the concept of calories in and calories out (burnt) as a means of weight loss and a strategy for avoiding fat intake to prevent ischemic heart disease and strokes. The public accepted this concept, and soon after, the industry came up with food products low in fats, replacing them with complex carbohydrates to make them palatable.

Then, the U.S. Department of Agriculture and the U.S. Department of Health and Human Services produced the Food Guide Pyramid, which guides **daily food choices.**

In it, they recommend serving the food products as follows:

- 6-11 servings in bread, cereal, rice, and pasta groups.
- 3-5 servings of the vegetable group.
- 2-4 servings of the fruit group.
- 2-3 servings of milk, yogurt, and cheese from the dairy group.
- 2-3 servings of the meat, poultry, fish, dry beans, egg, and nuts group
- Use sparingly fats, oils, and sweets.

Instead of improving health, all these measures and the opportunistic industry created the obesity pandemic. Seventy percent of the population today are overweight or obese, including children.

It is essential to clarify that obesity is not a weakness or lack of will by the overweight; it is a product of misinformation and ingrained habits of several generations that have contributed to the problem. It is time to demonize the obesity stigma often perpetuated with advice like stop eating so much; all that is needed is willpower.

What is needed is to fight the advertising for processed foods rich in sugars, avoid all these products, and replace snacks like potato chips, corn chips, and white bread with natural whole ingredients prepared at home.

Sugary products, when absorbed and present in the blood, stimulate the same brain receptors addictive drugs use, potentially creating a sugar addiction. (Wiss, Avena, & Pedro, 2018)

The **World Health Organization** (World Health Organization 2021) published a fact sheet on Obesity and overweight, which stated that worldwide obesity has tripled since 1975; it is a phenomenon that affects adults and children, including those under five years of age. They define being overweight for adults as having a BMI (Body Mass Index) equal to or greater than 25 and obesity with a BMI of 30 or greater. For children under five, being overweight is two standard deviations of the child growth standard median for the age, and obesity is three standard deviations. Similarly, the overweight parameter for children aged 5 to 19 is one standard deviation of the WHO of the growth reference median and two standard deviations for obesity. From 1975 to 2016, the number of overweight people has tripled, and for children has quadrupled.

Consequences of this problem (increased BMI, obesity) include type 2 diabetes, retinal damage, increased cardiovascular diseases, strokes, musculoskeletal disorders, especially osteoarthritis, a disabling degeneration of the joints from excess weight stress.

Cancers have become common, such as uterine, breast, prostate, liver, gallbladder, kidney, and colon.

The obesity pandemic has been widely publicized in the media worldwide. Two theories have been proposed: (1) a sedentary lifestyle and (2) the variety and ease of inexpensive palatable processed foods (World Health Organization 2021). It is most likely a combination of both.

Examples of a sedentary lifestyle include sedentary office work and air-conditioned and centrally heated spaces at work and home, significantly decreasing the BMR (Basal Metabolic Rate). The average body temperature has dropped 1°F in the last 150 years (Protsiv Myroslava,

2020). Regulating body temperature uses about 1000 calories a day. Burning 1000 calories with exercise is possible but not necessarily easy. Walking requires 20,000 to 25,000 steps, which takes about 2-3 hours. Running will need 1 ½ hours of running, not jogging.

Calorie restriction:

The concept of calorie restriction to combat obesity or overweight is not without merit. Dana G. Smith recently wrote in the New York Times (Smith, 2024), an article titled Could Eating Less Help You Live Longer?

It mentions experimental studies in animals reducing caloric intake by 30-40%, showing that several species of animals will live 30% longer. It is tough to prove the same in humans for multiple reasons, including the fact that the life span is much longer, the population is not as homogeneous as testing animal species explicitly developed for testing, and controlling the diet in humans is extremely difficult.

Why eating less would increase longevity? Multiple theories are trying to explain this phenomenon; the evolutionary process of all species indicates that wild animals, even today, go through periods of fasting while searching for food, including human ancestors. Even though life expectancy in those days was shorter, progress in medicine and the management of illnesses improved longevity to today's standards. The fact remains that obesity and obesity-related illnesses rob about 14 years of their lives. (NIH News releases, 2014).

Changing the metabolic Health.

Dieting and fasting for short periods (intermittent fasting) may change:

a) the metabolic health, relying less on glucose as an energy source and using other sources of energy, including other macronutrients (fat and protein); b) the destruction of damaged cells and tissues (apoptosis), the removal of the dead cells and tissues (autophagia), and the replacement of them with new cells and tissues.

A source of confusion is that not all tissues weigh the same; muscle (protein) is heavier than fat, but the caloric content of fat is twice that of muscle per gram.

Nevertheless, dieting and weight control associated with moderate exercise make you feel better and improve your metabolic health.

Does exercise help to lose weight?

The relationship between exercise and weight loss is unclear, complicated by the hypothesis of ***Constrained total energy expenditure*** (cyafitness.com, 2024) which states that exercise may not substantially increase calorie expenditure because of a reduced post-exercise energy expenditure. There are many critics of this hypothesis, primarily that it is based on observational data instead of double-blind studies. The issue remains that it is tough to do a long-term study about controlled diet and controlled-measured exercise type of study.

At the risk of repeating myself, moderate exercise makes you feel better, and a diet that can be integrated into your lifestyle will eventually produce weight loss.

Why do we eat?

We eat to produce energy for all body cells, organs, and systems to function, such as the respiratory system, which provides oxygen; the circulatory system, which distributes this oxygen; and the digestive system, which provides the source of energy. The amount of energy necessary for these functions is called the Basal Metabolic Rate (BMR). If we do any form of exercise, from simply walking to extreme exercises, the energy utilized will increase proportionally.

Our food contains macronutrients (Carbohydrates, proteins, fats, or lipids) and micronutrients (minerals, vitamins, and tissue protectors like antioxidants). The macronutrients cannot be absorbed as eaten; they need to be broken down into basic units through enzymes. Carbohydrates are broken down into monosaccharides, glucose, maltose, and fructose, and Proteins into amino acids. Fats can be absorbed as complex triglycerides by arranging themselves in Chylomicrons, groups of fatty acids combined with glycerol; this happens because fat is not soluble in water. It passes from the mucosa of the intestines to the lymphatics, bypasses the liver, and enters the blood circulation in the veins of the chest.

Digestion, absorption, and storage of all these macronutrients use energy, with carbs requiring the least energy for these processes and proteins requiring the most. **This is called the thermic effect of nutrients and means that your body burns more calories with a low-carb and high-protein diet.**

The thermic effect of fats is 3%, carbohydrates 7-10%, proteins 25-30%, and alcohol 15%.

Cell Respiration: What are the metabolic changes that eating produces?

As soon as you eat something, your body starts making changes through hormones and enzymes to convert what you eat into energy so all the cells and tissues can use this energy for the cell's functions and survival. (Krampf, 2019). This process of converting food into energy is called Cell Respiration. The chemical reactions necessary to produce and transport this energy are called metabolism.

The hormone that signals our body that food is coming is **Insulin,** produced by the pancreas in response to various stimuli, like a sweet taste in the mouth (sugar or substitutes) or when sugars get to the duodenum (first portion of the small bowel) stimulates the pancreas and produces insulin and pancreatic juice to break down the carbs and other macro-nutrients we ate. As carbohydrates are absorbed, blood sugar levels rise. The more often we eat or snack, the more the body responds to producing more insulin. If the body does not need extra energy to maintain normal function, then the insulin will signal to store the energy for the future. The extra energy may be stored as glycogen (a complex carbohydrate stored in the liver and muscle), as fat in subcutaneous tissue, or as visceral fat. There is no storage for proteins.

Glycogen is for immediate release when needed, like food in your refrigerator. The body will use fat to produce energy when glycogen storage has been exhausted. Body fat is not for immediate release, like food in your freezer. So, if one is overweight or obese and wishes to lose weight, one needs to consume the immediate-release energy and not eat yet to allow the burning of the stored fat.

Insulin has other functions besides signaling that food is coming. The **primary function** is to regulate the level of glucose (sugar) in the blood, so if we eat, especially carbohydrates frequently, the blood sugar will rise and spike and stimulate more production of insulin that will lower the glucose and store it as fat, this will happen when the glycogen storage places are already full. Therefore, insulin is a lipogenic hormone (which favors fat accumulation) that channels the energy to be stored as fat. In addition, lowering the glucose will make you hungry, so you eat again, and the cycle persists. Eventually, the organs will not respond typically to the high level of insulin, and insulin resistance will occur and produce type 2 diabetes.

All macronutrients have a two-step metabolism. The first or earliest set of chemical reactions (pathways) does not use oxygen and produces a modest amount of energy. The primary function of this early phase is to prepare the compounds to enter the second phase (**intermediate compounds**), where oxygen is used and produces large amounts of energy. The first phase is called **anaerobic pathways** (without oxygen), and the second is called **aerobic pathways** (with oxygen).

The first phase, the anaerobic pathway, occurs in the cytoplasm of the cells; for carbohydrates, it is called glycolysis; for fats, it is called lipolysis; and for proteins, proteolysis. They all produce similar compounds (intermediate compounds) that will enter the second phase or aerobic metabolism. That compound is often a 2-carbon attached to a co-enzyme called **Acetyl—CoA**. Intermediate compounds of carbs and fats are used for energy production, utilization, and storage. The intermediate compounds from proteins are used primarily to form new proteins for multiple uses, including the replacement of decaying tissues like hair, nails, skin, and linings of organs such as intestines, respiratory organs like bronchus and alveoli of the lungs, as well as apoptosis, or replacing damaged cell like post-exercise muscle cells.

The second phase, the aerobic Pathway, also called **The Krebs cycle or citric cycle**, is formed by a series of compounds from carbohydrates that, as they change, produce energy stored as chemical energy in the bonds of compounds named ATP (adenosine-an amino acid- and phosphorus). The presence of **insulin facilitates the entry of intermediate products from the anaerobic phase to the second phase, the aerobic phase**.

All these chemical reactions are called Metabolism, and these concepts are summarized in the following Flow Charts.

Flow Charts of Metabolic Pathways

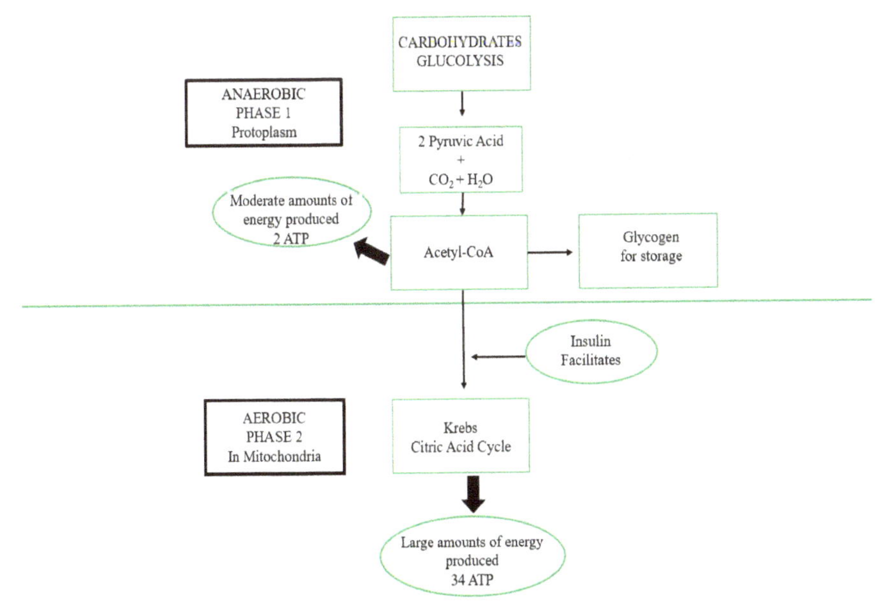

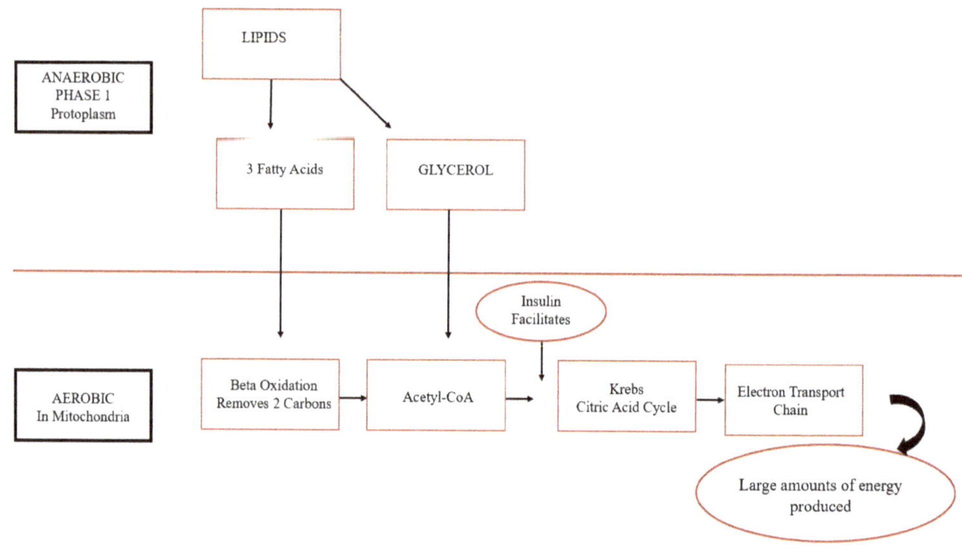

ANAEROBIC PHASE 1 Protoplasm
LIPIDS
3 Fatty Acids
GLYCEROL
Insulin Facilitates
AEROBIC In Mitochondria
Beta Oxidation Removes 2 Carbons
Acetyl-CoA
Krebs Citric Acid Cycle
Electron Transport Chain
Large amounts of energy produced

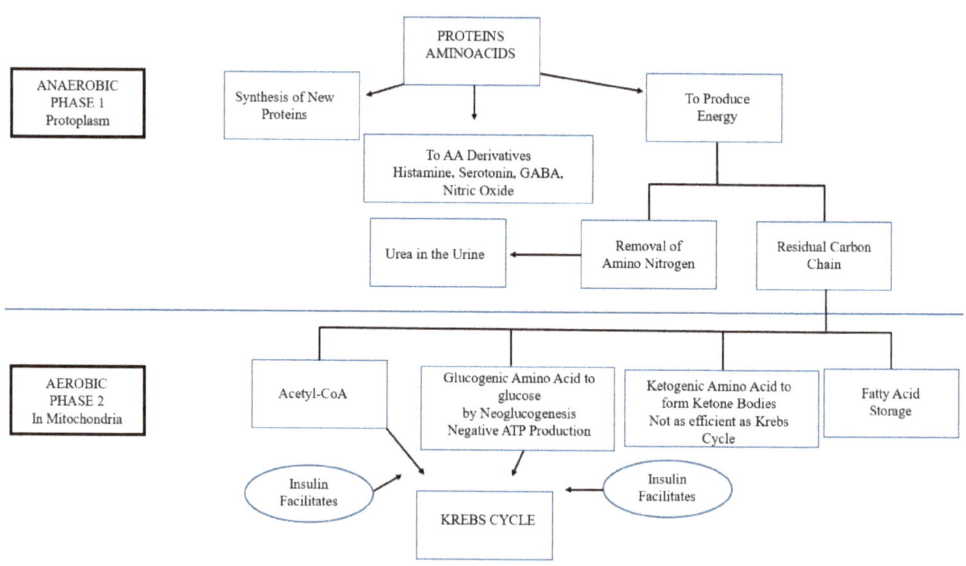

PROTEINS AMINOACIDS
ANAEROBIC PHASE 1 Protoplasm
Synthesis of New Proteins
To Produce Energy
To AA Derivatives Histamine, Serotonin, GABA, Nitric Oxide
Urea in the Urine
Removal of Amino Nitrogen
Residual Carbon Chain
AEROBIC PHASE 2 In Mitochondria
Acetyl-CoA
Glucogenic Amino Acid to glucose by Neoglucogenesis Negative ATP Production
Ketogenic Amino Acid to form Ketone Bodies Not as efficient as Krebs Cycle
Fatty Acid Storage
Insulin Facilitates
Insulin Facilitates
KREBS CYCLE

The diagram below shows in a more detailed form how the amino acid carbon skeletons enter the Krebs cycle.

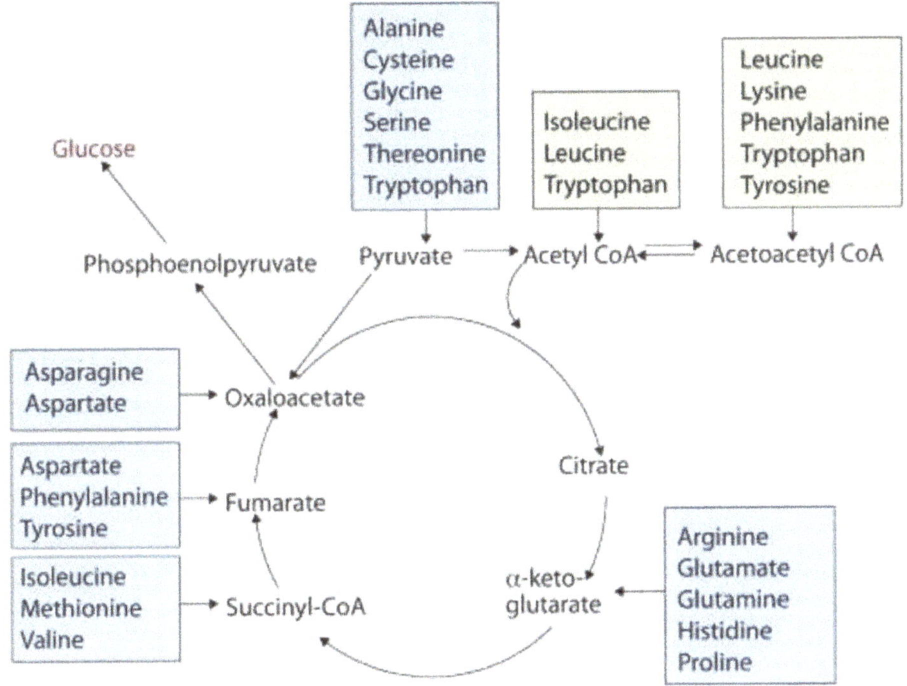

As you can see, the pathways the nutrients follow to produce the energy needed are very complex. Suffice it to say that there are two stages for the metabolism: 1) Anaerobic, which primarily prepares the intermediate compounds to enter the second phase, with a modest amount of energy produced, and 2) Aerobic or Krebs cycle, accepts the intermediate compounds and produces large amounts of energy. All of this is regulated through hormones.

In addition to Insulin signaling intracellular energy abundance, it facilitates the entry of the byproducts from the first phase of metabolism into high energy-producing pathways (aerobic) by **enhancing the irreversible conversion of pyruvate to Acetyl Co-A.** Acetyl-CoA then may be directly oxidized via the Krebs cycle or used for **fatty acid**

synthesis (lipogenesis) or enter **the ketogenesis pathway** with the formation of ketone bodies. A **low level of insulin** by a keto diet or a low to no carb diet and fasting slow the entry of acetyl Co-A into the high energy production of the Krebs or Citric acid cycle producer of multiple high energy compounds. Instead, it forms ketone compounds with lower energy production using more fatty acids to satisfy the body's needs. The ketone bodies cross the brain barrier, allowing the brain to use them for energy production (manifesting itself as alertness and sharp thinking despite fasting).

On the other hand, if there **is an excess of carbohydrates**, with all energy needs met, the Krebs cycle becomes extremely busy, exceeding its capacity. All the intermediate compounds of the Krebs cycle become fully occupied, and the entry of Acetyl CoA is slowed and will go to lipogenesis (formation of fat) **for storage**.

Therefore, excess carbohydrates, by stimulating insulin production and thus stimulating the activity of the aerobic pathways, will favor fat storage; think of insulin as a lipogenic hormone (favors the accumulation of fatty tissues).

All these chemical reactions we have discussed are the phase of catabolism, which breaks down the nutrients to be absorbed, utilized, and stored.

How is this this energy used?

First is the **Phase of Anabolism, which utilizes energy to form new cells to replace damaged ones. The damage may be caused by aging, like replacing skin layers daily, by trauma, like forming scars to heal trauma-damaged cells, replacing cell membranes, etc. Then,** energy is utilized for activities like breathing, the heart muscle pumping the blood, carrying oxygen to all tissues, maintaining the body temperature, etc.

Moreover, it is utilized for physical activity, like walking, manual tasks, and exercise.

What happens if you maintain a low level of insulin

All we have talked about in the previous paragraph is facilitated by the presence of high levels of insulin, facilitating the production of acetyl CoA, and the entry of the Acetyl-CoA into the Krebs cycle with the consequent production of large amounts of energy and accumulation of fatty tissue from the excess energy produced.

If one eats nearly no carbs, the insulin levels will remain low. This will slow the entry of the intermediate compounds into the Krebs cycle and favor the metabolism of the fatty tissues to form ketone bodies, which are not as efficient in producing energy. Because our organism is susceptible to low blood sugar, it will direct some energy to neo-glucogenesis (formation of blood sugar from fat or proteins). The energy used to produce this new glucose is larger than the energy produced by the metabolism of it.

This is often called **the switch to burn fat**; the Randal cycle stipulates that the more abundant nutrient, glucose (from carbs) or fatty acids (from fats), will direct the metabolism.

The Keto diet is based on this concept, but if excess calories are ingested, you will still accumulate fat to store excess energy.

Can metabolism be altered?

Several factors change our metabolism throughout our lives; they include:

 During childhood, much energy is utilized in growing up, making new tissues (muscle, skin, bones, etc.), and physical activity is abundant. A newborn will gain about an ounce daily during the first three months. Then, while young, we have proportionally more muscle mass; muscle is metabolically more active than other tissues like bone or fat. As we age, we lose muscle and get replaced by fat; therefore, our basal metabolic rate drops.

What we eat influences our metabolism. All nutrients have a **thermic effect**, which is the amount of energy necessary to utilize the nutrients, to be broken down, and to be absorbed and used for energy or storage. The sugars have the second lowest thermic effect ±7-10% (fats have the lowest 3%), and proteins have the highest (25-30%). So, a ***diet with limited carbs and protein richness will consume the most energy***. Additionally, alcohol produces seven calories per gram; they are utilized in a mandatory way, and the thermic effect is about 15%; alcohol consumption will lower the utilization of other nutrients, increasing fat storage.

How is Hunger produced and regulated?

The sensation of being hungry or satisfied during the interval between meals results from a balance between the hunger and satiety hormones. Disruption of this balance produces obesity or anorexia.

1. The usual mechanism of **satiety** (not being hungry) is mediated through hormones, such as **Leptin,** produced by the white fat cells. Leptin resistance will produce obesity, and **adiponectin is** produced by the same white fat cells, which has a role in energy production and metabolic processes (by increasing insulin release from the pancreas and accelerating insulin signaling in the liver and skeletal muscles. It also enhances glucose uptake in fat tissues); a low level of adiponectin is associated with obesity, type II diabetes, and the metabolic syndrome that accompanies type II diabetes and obesity. This may happen by **regulating sensitivity to Insulin (Sivapalan, 2022). It also has anti-inflammatory properties.**

Peptide YY:

It is secreted in response to fat and protein ingestion and produced in the distal small bowel. It has an anorectic effect, producing satiety by modulating neuronal activity in the lower brain (Efthimia Karra, 2009). This occurs by blocking the receptors for **neurotransmitters.** These neurotransmitters produce hunger and shorten the time between meals.

Cholecystokinin responds to dietary fat ingestion; it stimulates your gallbladder to contract and release bile into the intestine to break down fats and proteins. It stimulates the pancreas to release enzymes and suppresses gastric emptying to give time for its digestion to be completed, suppressing your appetite, giving the sensation of a full stomach, and inhibiting the production of the hunger hormone **Ghrelin**. It also triggers motility of the intestines, moving the intestinal contents along.

2. The **sensation of hunger** is induced **by low glucose in the blood, high insulin levels** (Loh Kim, 2017), and Ghrelin, or hunger hormone. It is produced in the stomach through baroreceptors that measure the pressure inside it. When pressure is low, Ghrelin is produced. This hormone peaks at our usual breakfast, lunch, and dinner times and bottoms at the postprandial period. This suggests that it is a learned response to existing habits.

This hormone, Ghrelin, has multiple functions, some direct and some indirect, through other hormones.

- Increases food intake and helps your body store fat by signaling the Hypothalamus (part of your brain) to increase appetite.
- **Helps trigger your <u>pituitary gland</u> to release growth hormone.** This protects your muscles from weakness and promotes bone formation and bone metabolism.
- Stimulates the transit of food through the digestive system, decreasing the production of the satiety hormones (leptin, adiponectin, polypeptide YY, and cholecystokinin).
- Plays a role in controlling blood sugars by producing hunger and how your body releases *insulin* (the hormone responsible for processing sugar).
- Certain genetic conditions and stress may promote accelerated obesity in specialized and specific locations (Hypothalamus)

through NPY neurons (neuro polypeptide sensitive neurons). (Chin, 2019)

As mentioned before, the counter-regulating hormone to Ghrelin is called Leptin. It is produced by the fatty tissues and encoded by the obese (ob.) gen. Leptin gives you the sensation of being full (satiety); its primary function is to regulate your long-term weight by serving as a marker of long-term energy stores (fat storage) for the central nervous system.

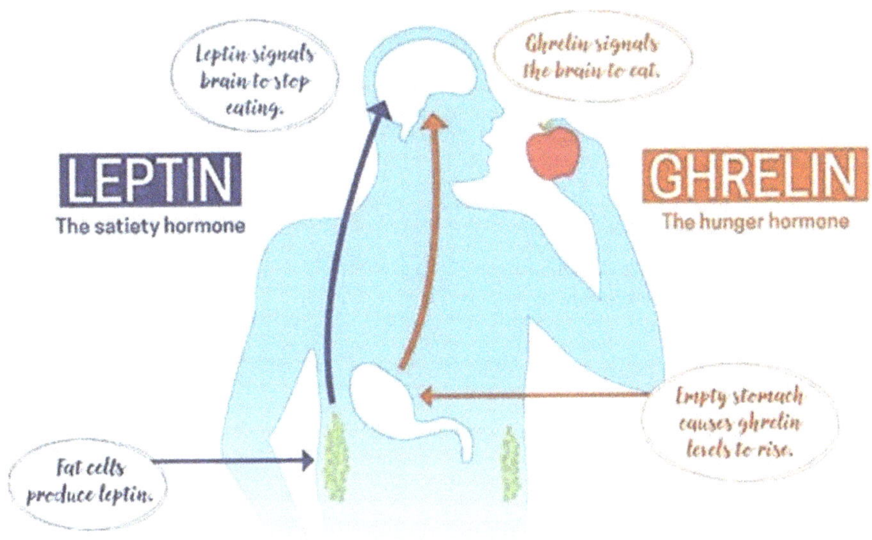

Credit for the diagram to weightwatchers.com. (WeightWatchers, 2019)

The **PYY gene encodes the peptide YY (PYY)**. It is released from the L cells in the ileum (distal small intestine) and colon (large intestine) and induces satiety, making you feel full. It has an ileal brake effect, decreases gastric emptying and pancreatic secretion, and slows gastrointestinal motility. The PYY concentration increases postprandially and decreases with fasting. Eating fiber-rich foods like fruits and vegetables increases the production of PPY because it increases the bulk of the intestinal contents. It, in a way, lets your brain know that digestion of the ingested nutrients is completed, **controlling the in-between meal period**.

Other peptides produced by the L cell of the intestines, such as GLP-1 (glucagon-like peptide), are used to treat Type II Diabetes for its positive effect on the alpha cells of the pancreas (the producer of Insulin) and associated weight loss. Recently, the FDA has been investigating several side effects of these drugs.

Table with information on Ghrelin and Leptin

Ghrelin	Leptin
Increases Appetite	Lowers Appetite
Location	Location
X cells of the Stomach	White adipose Cells
Target cells	Target Cells
Lateral Hypothalamic Brain cells (lower brain)	Ventromedial Hypothalamic Brain Cells (lower brain)
Action	Action
Hunger, ↑gastric motility, ↑gastric acid	Satiety
Inducers	Inducers
Hypoglycemia, low body weight	Insulin
Inhibitors	Inhibitors
Stomach Distension	Short-term fasting

(Weight 2019)

Other hormones that play a role in the regulation of metabolism.

Insulin Counter Hormones

Insulin counter-regulatory hormones such as adrenalin, cortisol, glucagon, and growth hormones are regulated through low blood sugar levels, which stimulate the secretion of these hormones. Adrenaline increases the Basic Metabolic rate, burning more energy. Growth hormone promotes lean mass maintenance and growth (muscles and bone). Cortisol, the fight or flee hormone, gives the sensation of well-being and energizes you, stimulating neo-glucogenesis (formation of glucose from proteins and glycerol from fats).

These counter-regulatory hormones oppose insulin effects; they have the opposite effects.

Disruptors of the average balance between Ghrelin and Leptin:
- **Lack of sleep: A single night of not getting** enough sleep will increase Ghrelin levels and lower Leptin levels. Thus, getting a good night's sleep is essential for weight control.
- **Chronic stress** elevates Ghrelin.
- **The types of food, such as** fatty foods and those high in sugars (like processed foods), elevate ghrelin and lower leptin, which may be a factor in the obesity epidemic.

If we have a breakfast composed primarily of carbohydrates (refined sugars and refined wheat flour are the worst), the cycle of high blood glucose in the blood - insulin secretion – low blood sugar – hunger will occur, and we will be hungry again in a couple of hours.

This has not been publicized enough in the past. The opposite has been recommended, like avoiding fats and animal meats because of their high-fat content. Therefore, fat was replaced by complex carbohydrates in low-fat processed foods. In addition, public information, beginning with the food pyramid and now the "my plate," eating multiple small meals throughout the day and counting calories, **has led us to the overweight–obesity epidemic.**

Public behavior from the days of early post-World War II, when three square meals a day, no snacking, and no obesity (World Health Organization 2021), to today, with decreased consumption of meats and fat, counting calories, and multiple snacking, produced the obesity epidemic. We are doing something wrong. We are stimulating hunger by inhibiting the production of satiety hormones (YY peptide and cholecystokinin), promoting multiple small meals a day, and counting calories to match the basal metabolic rate.

The Basal Metabolic Rate is the amount of energy (calories) necessary for the cells of our body to stay alive, tissues to fulfill their function, and organs and systems to do the same: the heart to beat, the nervous system to command what we do, digestive system to process and absorb the nutrients, etc. This basal metabolic rate adjusts to what fuel is provided; it will slow down if enough calories are not provided.

Counting calories and restricting their intake to somewhat less than the basal metabolic rate presumes that the metabolic rate does not change. All studies of calorie-counting diets have demonstrated that it does not work; either weight is not lost or is regained in short order. Additionally, a reduced or deficient caloric diet (counting calories) makes our organisms lower our basal metabolic rate, reduces fuel utilization, converts a Cadillac into a Fiat 500, and does not reduce hunger.

As mentioned before, regulating blood sugar levels is critical, mainly because the risk of low blood sugar is significant because of potential neurological damage. Nature has placed a safety mechanism; it will protect us from neurological damage even when fasting for prolonged periods.

This mechanism is through the so-called Cycle of Randle, where the balance of the two substrates, glucose from carbohydrates and free fatty acids from fats. This cycle will use the more dominant substrate for energy production; for example, if one is fasting for extended periods, the blood sugar will remain within normal limits (80-120mg/dl) by utilizing fatty acids for energy production, either from dietary intake or from fatty storages. Conversely, if glucose is abundant, it will be used for energy production (from insulin production) and store the fatty acids as subcutaneous fat. This is the so-called switch to burn fat, like on the Keto diet.

Losing Weight

To lose weight, reshape our bodies to lower fat storage, and increase lean mass, it is necessary to control hunger by lowering insulin levels, decreasing the production of ghrelin, facilitating the production of leptin and Peptide YY, and increasing physical activity to gain lean weight and allow the Insulin counter hormones do their job.

Low Carb or no Carb diet

A low-carb or no-carb diet will decrease the production of insulin by moderating the glucose level in the blood and, therefore, not stimulating the production of Insulin. The production of ghrelin is more challenging to control. However, studies show that fasting for periods does not increase ghrelin levels after a time, and intermittent fasting for an extended period decreases it. A diet rich in fiber is filling (produces satiety) and will keep hunger under control. The increase in physical activity does not need to be excessive and will vary with the individual's age and capacity for exercise. Walking or light gymnastics suffice, allowing for increased lean mass and reduced body fat content; it is unnecessary to get to a lactic acidosis state other than for conditioning.

Whatever we eat, carbohydrates, proteins, or fats eventually get broken down by a pathway that does not use oxygen into a molecule called Acetyl Coenzyme A or **Acetyl-CoA** (or similar intermediate compounds) that are the primary fuel to produce energy through the aerobic pathways. If all energy requirements are met, it will go to storage as fat.

As discussed, food uses several pathways to produce energy and maintain the Basal Metabolic rate (BMR). The initial process for all the types of macronutrients is **anaerobic,** meaning it does not use oxygen. The energy produced is transported for utilization or storage through compounds containing phosphorus and an amino acid, adenosine.

This process is called glycolysis for carbs (it produces 4 ATPs but uses 2 ATPs, so its net production is 2 ATPs), proteolysis for proteins, and lipolysis for lipids.

These anaerobic pathways produce a modest amount of energy; as mentioned before, this energy is carried to all cells by molecules that contain phosphorus. The energy is held in the several connections of Phosphorus to an amino acid (adenosine). There are three types of these compounds, depending on the number of connections with phosphorus, established: AMP (one), ADP (two), and ATP (three). How many ATPs are produced depends on the type of macronutrient being metabolized; in addition to this modest amount of energy produced by the anaerobic pathways, residual compounds (intermediate compounds) such as **Acetyl CoA**, a 2-carbon compound.

These compounds will enter the **aerobic pathways** (stimulated by the presence of insulin) and produce abundant amounts of energy and two molecules of CO2 in the case of glucose (glucose is how the carbs are absorbed), and the fatty acids have many more carbons. Not all the fatty acids are the same length, so the energy produced will vary. Proteins are rarely used for energy production, but in starvation, the amino acids will be used to produce energy; they also have different length chains of carbons, so their energy production will vary. The use of amino acids for energy production will produce muscle mass loss.

Under normal circumstances, where all the energy needs are covered, and no excess energy is ingested (BMR + activity energy), the energy produced is summarized as follows:

Anaerobic Pathways: The macronutrients are absorbed in the simplest form possible, enter the bloodstream, and are transported to the body's chemical plant, the liver.

- **Glucose,** by glycolysis, will produce 2 Acetyl CoA and 2 CO_2; it will also produce 2 NADH2 (similar function as ATPS) and 2 ATPs, which will later enter the electron transport cycle.
- **Triglycerides (fats)**will be broken into glycerol (which goes to form glucose) and fatty acids. The fatty acids

produced by beta-oxidation will produce Acetyl CoA, 1 NADH2, and 1 FADH2 (the latter of which will enter the electron transport cycle) for each of the two carbons. The residual fatty acid will reenter the Beta oxidation cycle, losing two carbons and producing the same compounds as in the first pass. These steps will repeat until no carbon is left in the residual fatty acid.

- **Amino acids (proteins)** are usually not used to produce energy but are mainly used to repair damaged proteins in the cells or replace damaged cells. However, they may be used for energy during starvation or when excess dietary proteins are ingested. The carbon chain in the amino acids varies in length (number of carbons); therefore, the energy produced will vary. Their catabolism will produce Acetyl CoA or other intermediate compounds. The diagrams shown before during the discussion of metabolism illustrate the different intermediate compounds and their site of entry into the aerobic phase *Flow Charts of Metabolic Pathways*. The purpose of sharing these flow charts is to show the complexity of the metabolic pathways.

Aerobic pathways:

Since all macronutrients end up as Acetyl CoA or similar intermediate compounds, they can enter the Krebs Cycle or Citric Acid Cycle and its associated electron transport chain to produce abundant energy (Google Classroom, 2024). Each molecule of **Acetyl Co A** will produce 12 ATP;

each NADH$_2$ will produce an average of 3 ATPs, and FADH$_2$ will produce 1 ATP. So, a Glucose molecule produces 2 Acetyl CoA 12 ATPs in the Krebs cycle plus six from the NADH and two from the FADH from the initial glycolysis for a total of 32 ATPs. The long chains of carbons of the lipids produce similar amounts of energy products for each of the two carbons, so it is a much denser macronutrient than carbs.

Low Carb Diet

To understand how the low-carb diet works, it is only necessary to **remember that there are 2 phases to produce energy: anaerobic and aerobic; insulin levels regulate how much energy is produced by modulating the entry of acetyl CoA or other intermediate compounds into the second phase. Hunger can be altered by the type of macronutrients we eat (fiber-rich carbs), proteins (preferably plant-based), and fats preferably unsaturated.**

A table summarizing the energy production by the elements of metabolism is discussed below.

Table of nutrients and metabolic compounds and energy production.

Nutrient	Kcal/ g.	Kcal/mol g.	Mol mass	ATP prod. Anaerobic	ATP trough Krebs	What are they?		
ATP	12		241g.			Energy carrier		
Glucose	4.5	456	180g.	2	48	The byproduct of carbs		
Fat(palmitic) saturated fat 16 C chain	9.0	1548	256.4	27-2= 25 3 ATPs for each 2 carbons	128 per palmitic acid 16 ATP per each Acetyl CoA	The most common Fatty acid		
Protein	45	variable	Eg.18000	variable		All muscles	Become amino acids	
Pyruvate to Acetyl-CoA					3ATPs equivalents (2NADH)	Potentially from all Macronutrients	Entry point to the Krebs cycle.	
Ketogenic amino acid	Ketogenesis			22ATPs	Variable depending on the length of the carbon chain	Low insulin or high fatty acids induce ketogenesis	Low Insulin decreases the enzyme lipase	Low lipase increases fatty acids.
Glucogenic amino acid	Gluconeogenesis in balance (energy loss) uses 9 ATP equivalents.			2 ATPs	2 ATPs 2NADH(3ATPs) 2Acetyl-CoA	To maintain blood sugars in prolonged fasting		

Deeds required for Weight loss.

What we want to achieve while dieting is:

Hunger control.

1. The sensation of hunger is said to come from hypoglycemia, low blood glucose, and ghrelin produced by the stomach when the gastric pressure is low.

   If the feeding is frequent and contains simple carbs, the yo-yo effect of snacking and frequent eating will produce glucose spikes. Your body's response will have the pancreas produce insulin to lower the high glucose, and when it is down, you become hungry again, and the cycle repeats. If this continues for long periods, **Insulin resistance** develops, and you become Pre-Diabetic and later a type 2 Diabetic.

   To avoid this, it is necessary to avoid blood sugar peaks and limit the carbohydrates responsible for them.

   A low-carb, no-carb, or keto diet (low-carb and high-fat) will accomplish this. The keto diet has the disadvantage of high fat intake, which, when sustained for prolonged periods, will eventually increase the risk of increased cholesterol of low density (LDL) with the associated increased risk of cardiovascular diseases. Additionally, fats have a low thermic effect (3%) and contribute the highest caloric content, 9 Calories per gram.

The circadian rhythm of ghrelin (hunger hormone) production at customary breakfast, lunch, and dinner time suggests that it may be a learned cycle. This is further suggested by the decrease in ghrelin production with intermittent fasting. An attempt to modify the production of ghrelin is made through a form of bariatric surgery with sleeve resection of part of the stomach, which is in part based on the observation in the late '50s and early sixties that patients who had Gastric resections for peptic ulcer disease had significant permanent weight loss.

A counter-hormone to Ghrelin, **Leptin** is produced by the adipose tissue and encoded by the obese (OB.) gene.

2. Lower insulin levels by avoiding sugary foods and drinks, processed carbs like products from white flowers, and fiber-rich food to delay stomach emptying, decrease the production of Ghrelin, and increase the production of Peptide YY.

   - This will prevent or slow the entry of acetyl CoA into the Krebs cycle, increasing ketogenesis, a less efficient pathway because part of the ketone bodies will be lost through breathing, part through the urine, and the remaining will be metabolized through lower energy production.
   - This will double effect: 1) rump up gluconeogenesis to maintain glucose levels. This is inefficient because it takes more energy to create the new glucose than is produced by burning it. 2) It stimulates the secretion of counter-regulating hormones as the glucose falls; they maintain the

BMR by adrenalin and epinephrin, increasing the heart rate and blood pressure and consuming more energy. The glucagon increases gluconeogenesis, and the growth hormone increases lean mass.

- The production of the insulin-counter-regulating hormones follows a sequential pattern: the insulin level drops; if it continues, then glucagon will act; if glucose still falls, then epinephrin and norepinephrine will rise; if glucose continues to fall, growth hormone will rise; if glucose continues to fall, then cortisol will increase, and if glucose keeps on falling, then coma will occur in diabetic people.

Develop habits that are helpful to control hunger.

3. Awareness of eating patterns: slow down. (D'cruz, 2023)

   a) **Be aware of how you eat**. Pay attention to flavor and other sensations like the food's temperature and texture. Put your utensils down between bites. Learn to differentiate between physical hunger and emotional or boredom hunger. Take a deep breath and talk to other people at the table.

   b) **Be aware of your emotions and sensations**. Intermittently check how you feel: Are you hungry? Satisfied? Bloated? Learn how your body tells you that you are overeating. Each person's body responds differently; some perspire over their nose, some develop hick-ups, and others need to burp. Learn to eat to 80% full and then stop eating.

Should you include fasting in your diet plan?

Fasting has 3 phases.

- Phase 1 burns the storage of carbohydrates in your body, glycogen from the Liver and Muscle (refrigerator)
- Phase 2 burns the fat storage initially from skeletal fat; when near ideal weight is reached, you start burning visceral fat.
- Phase 3, when no fat is available, starts burning protein from the lean muscle, producing starvation.
- Clearly, one should avoid Phase 3, where a healthy body maintains lean muscle mass. Intermitting fasting uses phase 1 and may be extended into early phase 2.
- Phase one requires about 10 hours of fasting. I prefer skipping breakfast, so you will have the whole night to fast from when you finish dinner, maybe 7 or 8 p.m. Your first meal should be around 11 to 12 noon when you break your fast, allowing for about 4 hours of fat-burning.
- Pre-fast meals should stimulate the production of hormones that promote satiety, including leptin produced by the fatty tissues, polypeptide y-y by the distal small bowel, enzymes produced by the pancreas, and bile from the liver. Should include Proteins (*cheese, tofu, fish or seafood, skinless defatted poultry, eggs*), fiber (*beans and legumes, whole grains, vegetables, fruit*), and healthy fats (*avocado, olive oil, nuts*).

- During this period, your insulin remains low, and the aerobic pathways slow down because Insulin facilitates the byproducts from the anaerobic pathways to enter the aerobic pathways. A low insulin level slows this entry.

Fasting Metabolic changes: This fasting produces metabolic changes that occur sequentially.

After you have had a meal, the first change is a spike in blood sugar, particularly if you have had a carb-rich meal. Your body responds to this by producing insulin that will decrease glucose. During this stage, your body utilizes stored glycogen (refrigerator storage). If the fasting is prolonged enough and all the glycogen from the liver has been used, your body switches and starts using stored fat (the freezer storage). This transition happens because the insulin levels drop, allowing the fat cells to release stored fatty acids. These fatty acids are then converted in the liver to ketone bodies that can be used for energy production (the low Insulin levels slow the entry of intermediate compounds into the Krebs cycle, forcing the use of less efficient pathways). This metabolic shift has several benefits: **burning fat storage, improved insulin sensitivity, and cognitive benefits.** The time for these changes to occur varies for everyone; usually, a 14-hour fast will go through the consumption of stored glycogen and the early fat-burning stage. One needs to find the optimal length of fasting for oneself, pay attention to the signals your body gives you, and adjust the length of fasting accordingly. A similar process occurs without intermittent fasting if you make your meals low in carbohydrates, mainly processed carbs like flour and bread, and eat fiber-rich carbs, which are allowed (not absorbed) about 15g of net carbs (total carbs minus fiber) per meal with three meals per day.

4. Use a less efficient metabolic path that burns the most fuel without producing excess energy. In other words, ensure our body functions like a big old Cadillac. You achieve this by burning fat during periods of ketosis. You reach ketosis after burning all the stored glycogen, usually achieved overnight. If you postpone breakfast, you will burn fat until you break your fast.

5. Intermittent fasting with no snacks and only two meals daily also works. Serial measurement of ghrelin in prolonged fasting shows a decreasing production level instead of a rise, so some recommend intermittent fasting to achieve this. This falls into the keto-diet recommended cycle of 16 hours of fasting and 8 hours a day for your meals and snacks. (Robillos, 2020)

6. Concerning using a less efficient pathway, if we could direct the traffic of Acetyl CoA to ketogenesis, then it would not enter the aerobic cycle of Krebs and would not produce as large an amount of energy. This is usually referred to as a state of ketosis, where your body primarily uses fat instead of glucose through a less efficient pathway that is not as efficient in producing energy, ideally using your fat **and not excessively ingested fats**. This is achieved with a no-carb diet and intermittent fasting. Eventually, non-refined carbs should be added when optimal weight is achieved. Instead, add complex carbs rich in fiber, primarily as fresh fruits and vegetables.

7. Make sure that it can be incorporated into your lifestyle.

Weight loss Benefits

In addition to the aesthetics of weight loss, there are immediately related benefits, such as alleviating joint problems from reduced stress from being overweight and decreased inflammation, with drops in the C-reactive protein levels an indicator of inflammation. Other benefits include the reversal of type 2 diabetes. (Ko, 2022 Jun 30; 31(2)) if no permanent damage has occurred to systems like renal failure, ocular retinal damage, and progressive CVD (Yancy, Foy, & all, 2005).

There is much talk about cholesterol levels and cardiovascular disease. Cholesterol is an essential lipid for protecting all cellular membranes; in the nervous system, it forms part of the myelin, a lipoprotein that envelops the axons (tails) of the neurons forming the nerves. It is also a precursor of androgens and estrogens.

Cholesterol from our diets represents about 20% of the total cholesterol content in our bodies; the remaining 80% is synthesized by liver cells. Cholesterol is transported in the blood (to where it will be utilized for the membranes of new cells) by lipoproteins of low-density LDL, very low-density VLDL (bad cholesterols), and High-density HDL, or good cholesterol.

The types of Transported cholesterol levels have been used for many years as decision-making indicators for treating patients with high risk of Cardiovascular events.

New compounds that may be more accurate in their predictive value have been found. They are called **ceramides** (Revuelta Soba, 2023), a small family of lipids formed by a sphingoid base (amino alcohol) combined with a fatty acid. More than a hundred of these ceramides have been identified in the skin.

It is apparent that they have a predictive value for cardiovascular diseases and a predictive value for progression of the same (Shalaby, Aidaros, & all, 2022), including cardiac-related mortality. There are many different ceramides. The ones with this predictive value are C16:0, C18:0, and C24:1. The first number is the number of carbons of the lipid acid, and the second number indicates the number of double bonds. The concentration of ceramides and similar compounds is high in the VLDL, therefore, the predictive value of VLDL (Mucinski, 2020).

This is still in the research process and unavailable for clinical use. (Shalaby 2021)

What are the benefits of fasting?

The most obvious benefit is weight loss, which, if done for extended periods, does not reach a plateau like most other diets. This is because it lowers insulin levels and increases insulin sensitivity.

- Has some advantages over diets, like it is simple, accessible, and convenient. When not fasting allows one to enjoy occasional life pleasures, it works with any diet. It is powerful, allowing for the cure of type 2 diabetes in some patients if type 2 diabetes has not created permanent damage.
- It improves mental clarity and concentration, avoiding the postprandial somnolence of a big meal and restoring the acuity of the periods between meals.

- Induces body fat loss in both subcutaneous and visceral fat.
- Lowers blood sugar levels and increases insulin sensitivity.
- Lowers blood cholesterol.
- Decreases inflammation.

  Many of these benefits are also common in diets that induce weight loss.

Reverses aging and prolongs life through apoptosis or programmed cellular death. When cells become dysfunctional, some cellular internal parts may be changed, but they must be replaced if the damage is too extensive. For this to occur, creating "space" (by autophagy) for the new healthy cells produced through the growth hormone's stimulation is necessary. This is a continuous process, so the "space" must constantly be created for the new cells, (Revuelta Soba, 2023).

- It may prevent Alzheimer's disease, again by autophagy, which cleans out the amyloid beta that otherwise accumulates in the brain cells of Alzheimer's patients.

It should be said that fasting is not for everyone, particularly in the extended modality where lean muscle mass loss occurs. Intermittent fasting by skipping one meal a day will accelerate weight loss without the loss of lean mass (muscle).

Diet Failures

All diets fail. The mode of failure varies from difficulty adhering to the diet to the plan being too complicated and challenging to incorporate into a lifestyle. Even the low-carb diets become challenging to continue for a long time. They all reach a plateau where weight cannot be lost any longer.

These failures make people abandon them. When you reach that plateau, it is time to add intermittent fasting to the plan because it is simple and is not doing anything, but doing less makes it possible to add it to your lifestyle. The duration of the fast period can be as simple as skipping a meal. I think the best one to skip is breakfast because it allows for 16-17 hours of fasting, from finishing dinner the night before until lunchtime.

The primary purpose of these diets should be to reduce insulin levels; this will channel the metabolic pathways to favor the entry of nutrients to less efficient pathways like the ketone bodies pathway and slow down the most efficient pathways like the aerobic Krebs cycle.

Low insulin levels with normal glucose levels also signal the need for counter-regulatory hormones (which have an opposite effect than Insulin): Glucagon, adrenalin, epinephrine, and growth hormone. These hormones maintain a high BMR (basal metabolic rate) and glucose at normal levels by gluconeogenesis, an energy-consuming process that promotes lean mass and bone growth.

Energy is essential for the survival and healthy replacement of cells and tissues, such as healing wounds and repairing muscle fibers damaged by exercise. Since it is not being obtained from glucose, it is replaced by the breakdown of fatty tissues, either subcutaneous or visceral, if ingested lipids **are not too abundant**.

At this point, regulatory mechanisms should be added to the list. In addition to hormonal regulation (Insulin and counter-regulatory hormones to insulin, like glucagon, epinephrin, nor-epinephrin, and growth hormone), there is another mechanism called the Randle cycle.

In 1963, the Medical Journal Lancet published an article by Phillip Randle. (Hue & Taegtmeyer, 2009). Proposing the regulation of pathways to produce energy by a nutrient-mediated cycle in which glucose and fatty acids compete for oxidation and energy production pathways. A high glucose inhibits the utilization of the fatty acids, and vice versa; a high concentration of fatty acids inhibits the utilization of glucose. This cycle is the basis for low-carb diets and keto diets.

Creating a Physiological Diet

To construct the appropriate Diet, we will review the must-haves. We will use our understanding of metabolism, pathways that nutrients follow, and how to manipulate the hormones that regulate these pathways to produce satiety and avoid hunger.

Weight loss Strategies:

Reduction of aerobic Metabolism

Reducing carbohydrate intake to 45g per day (15g per meal) as part of a low-carb diet can lead to a state called ketosis, where the body adapts to using fat for energy instead of glucose from carbohydrates (Randle cycle). This shift can reduce aerobic metabolism as the body relies more on fat as a fuel source. However, the exact reduction in aerobic metabolism can vary from person to person based on several factors, including physical activity level, overall health, how the body adapts to the diet, and particularly the individual's muscle mass (muscle uses more energy than fatty tissues).

It is important to note that while some experience reduced energy levels shortly after reducing carbs, others may find their energy levels remain stable or even increase after an adaptation period, particularly in organs that utilize ketone bodies like the brain and Heart). If you are considering such a diet, especially for athletic performance or health reasons, it is advisable to consult with a healthcare professional or a dietitian. They can provide personalized advice and meet your nutritional needs while following a low-carb diet.

On a diet of 2500 Calories daily, if you make it a low-carb version and obtain a 30% reduction of ATP production by reducing the aerobic metabolism, your actual caloric intake would be 1750 usable Calories. If your basal metabolism is 2500, you would have a caloric deficit of 750 calories, but you would have eaten enough to suppress hunger. It is sort of the best of both worlds.

- **Reduce Insulin levels**: It will decrease the conversion rate of Pyruvic acid (intermediate compound from anaerobic metabolism) to Acetyl CoA; the pyruvic acid then will convert into lactic acid or go to gluconeogenesis (energy expenditure high). This will prevent the entry of acetyl CoA into the Krebs cycle and will increase ketogenesis, a less efficient pathway because part of the ketone bodies formed will be excreted in the breath (apple breath odor) and in the urine; this is due to ketone bodies being water-soluble. The remaining is metabolized at a lower energy production.

- **Increase gluconeogenesis.** To maintain glucose levels at a normal range (low blood sugar is very damaging to the central nervous system), **gluconeogenesis will rump up,** burning additional energy since it consumes more energy than the energy produced by the breakdown of the glucose generated.

- *Increase production of Insulin Counter Hormones.* Low insulin with a lower glucose level will stimulate the secretion of the counter-regulatory hormones as the glucose level falls. The counter-regulatory hormones to insulin will maintain the BMR through adrenalin and norepinephrine, increasing the heart rate and blood pressure and consuming more energy. The **glucagon** increases gluconeogenesis since the carb storage is depleted. The **growth hormone** will promote lean mass growth, often producing a slowdown in weight loss because of a gain in the lean mass. It is better to go by waist size rather than weight during those periods.

- The sequence of production of counter-regulatory hormones follows a pattern. First, the insulin levels will decrease; if the glucose level keeps falling, the glucagon will increase. If glucose still falls, epinephrin and norepinephrine will rise; growth hormone will increase if the glucose level still falls. If glucose still falls, cortisol will increase; if this fails, the patient falls into a coma. This is the reason why when a diabetic patient comes to the emergency room in a coma, the first response is to give them glucose intravenously. (should it be eliminated? Is it repetitive?)

- *Ideal Diet.* A diet consisting of reduced carbs (15g of carbs per each of 2-3 meals a day is generally satisfactory), **abundant fibers** (leafy vegetables, pulses, and beans, konjac root products, broccoli, cauliflower), **abundant protein** (meats, fish, other seafood, eggs, Greek yogurt), and **adequate fat intake** will control hunger by reducing ghrelin production, increasing leptin production, and peptide YY contributing to hunger control.

- **Ideal Ingredients.** Food should be rich in fiber, soluble and insoluble, unsaturated fatty acids (rich in omega 3), and beta-sitosterol, all of which are linked to lowering LDL cholesterol. Examples include avocado, nuts and seeds, fish, especially salmon and tuna (mono to poly unsaturated ½ to ½), and olive oil in a mono to poly 9/1 ratio. Be aware of the calories in the serving size.
- **Accelerate catabolism.** Some products, such as green tea, capsaicin (chilis), and apple cider vinegar, can only enhance metabolic rate to a limited extent.

To succeed with our diet, it must be incorporated into our lifestyle. Eventually, you will make a lifestyle change for life.

Additionally, you must develop habits that will facilitate your adherence to the diet and avoid certain pitfalls.

Habits to develop:

Adopt Healthy eating habits. Some of these recommendations apply to the maintenance of weight diets.

- **Develop portion control:** To avoid calorie surplus, you must develop the habit of portion control. Divide your plate into three portions: ½ for vegetables cooked or salads, ¼ for proteins, and ¼ for starchy vegetables. The last ¼ (starchy vegetables) applies when you have achieved your ideal weight. During the weight-loss period, divide your plate into two halves for vegetables and proteins.

- **Be aware of how you eat:** Consider the flavor and other sensations like temperature and texture. Slow down, put your utensils down after each bite, take a deep breath, and talk to other people at the table.

- **Be aware of your emotions and sensations:** intermittently check how you feel: hungry, satisfied, or bloated. Learn how your body tells you overate. Each body responds differently; some perspire over their nose; others develop hiccups or need to burp. Learn to eat only to be 80% satisfied, then stop eating and double-check 15 minutes later; most likely, you will be satisfied.

- **Learn to differentiate** between physical hunger and emotional or boredom hunger.

- **Eat healthy, balanced meals that promote satiety. Include high-fiber foods like fruits, whole grains, vegetables, legumes, beans, nuts, and seeds. Move around after eating; if you are too full to do so,** you have had excess food. Avoid saturated fats in meats and dairy (butter, whole milk, cheese). Instead, use plant-based fats like guacamole, hummus, and almond butter. Make sure that the substitutes do not have added sugars or saturated fats.

Avoid Pitfalls.

- The first week or so, you may have withdrawal symptoms because of the addictive properties of sweets, as discussed previously (Roberts, 2021)

- Stay hydrated and drink water when hungry, just in case of confusing thirst for hunger.
- Consume fiber-rich foods like fruits, vegetables, whole grains, legumes, and beans.
- Incorporating healthy fats, like avocado, nuts and seeds, and olive oil, induces satiety by up to 20-35% of daily calories.
- Incorporate proteins; they induce satiety, and the best are plant-based proteins like legumes and beans. In addition, they increase muscle mass, and they burn more calories to eat and metabolize. Proteins improve the quality of aging by improving the biological age of all cells.
- Practice awareness when eating.
- Make sure your meals are balanced; they keep you full longer.
- Practice awareness of flavors, textures, temperatures, and eating enjoyment.
- Snacking for hunger control, e.g., fresh fruits, vegetables, hummus as a dip or instead of butter. Berries with Greek yogurt, vegetables with hummus, and unsalted nuts.
- Whole foods vs. processed foods. Avoid processed foods; whole foods have more fiber. Excretion studies show that whole foods excrete contain more residual calories than processed foods.

Social Meals

- Pre-plan social meals to avoid deviations.
- Choose the Restaurant yourself.
- Visit the Restaurant yourself, see the menu, and choose what you will eat before the social meal.

- Choose healthy options, such as low-carb, high-protein, and healthy fats.
- Choose lighter foods like fish, seafood, salads, and grilled vegetables.
- Eating alone is a missed opportunity.

A series of recipes for two or three meals a day will be offered. Choose the recipes with 15g. or less net carbs for weight loss. After reaching your ideal weight, you can use any of the recipes and replace some of the low-carbohydrate products like skinny noodles from konjac root instead of regular noodles, cauliflower rice for brown rice, and cauliflower pizza dough for flour dough, remembering to mind your serving portions.

Recipes for Weight Loss

Low-carbohydrate diets require abstinence from refined flour and sugars, which implies no bread, pastries, pasta, pizza dough, or taco shells. This is no easy task. Fortunately, substitutes exist in flours with a significant amount of fiber to modulate the absorption of the carbs and prevent spikes in blood sugar and insulin production.

Finished products with a low carbohydrate content can be easily found online. One downside of these products is their cost. Shredded cheeses are also available in packages; their cost is reasonable, but it is still best to shred your own because the pre-packaged shredded cheese contains added anti-caking compounds that, I believe, modify the taste and prevent it from melting properly.

Table 6: Nutrients in food of plants

COMPOSITION OF LOW CARB FRIENDLY FOODS

NAME	FAT	g/100g CARBS	g/100g DIGESTABLE CARB	g/100g PROTEIN	g/100g FIBER
Garlic		33.3	0	6.66	33.3
Avocados	15	8.5	0.6	2	7.9
Lettuce	0.28	3.09	1.12	1.16	1.97
Spinach		3.6	1.4	2.9	2.2
Radishes		4	1.6	0.8	2.4
Asparragus		3.7	1.9	2.2	1.8
zucchini		3.1	2.1	0.5	1
Celery		3	2.24	0.75	0.76
Mushrooms		3.28	2.28	3.14	1
Eggplant	0.1	4.8	2.4	0.8	2.4
Tomato		3.9	2.7	0.9	1.2
Cauliflower		5	3	2	2
Cabbage	0.1	5.2	3	1.1	2.2
Cucumber		4	3.4	0.3	0.6
Broccoli		6	3.6	2.5	2.4
Green Beans	0.2	7	4.3	1.8	2.7
Brussel sprouts		7.6	5.04	2.56	2.56
Jicama		10	5.1	0.75	4.9
Bell Peppers		10	7	1	3
Artichokes	0.4	14	7	3.5	7
Onion	0.2	10	7	1.43	3
Kale		12	9.4	4.4	2.6
Lentils		20	11.2	9	8.8
Brown rice		23	21.2	2.6	1.8
Beans		62	53.4	8.8	8.6
potatoes		20.1	18.3	1.9	1.8
parsnips		17.6	13.5	1.2	4.1

A low Carb diet should contain/24h period: 100 g of total carbs, (for keto <50g), 70 g of protein and enough fat to provide a total of 2000-2500 cal.

Table 7: Nutrients of food from the animal kingdom

Composition of proteins of animal origen

All Raw	g/100g Fat	g/100g Carb	g/100g Protein	g/100g Fiber	Kcal/100g Kcal.
Beef ground	11.8	0	26.1	0	214
Tenderloin	8.9	0	26	0	210
Sirloin cap	16.4	0	25.88	0	249
Eye Round	4.7	0	29.41	0	170
Chuck eye roast	8.47	0	27	0	183.5
Grouper	1.2	0	21.9	0	104
Flounder	2	0	14	0	80
Snapper	1.76	0	22.4	0	128
Monk Fish	1.7	0	16.4	0	86
Chicken Breast	3.6	0	31	0	165
Chicken Thigh	3.9	0	18.8	0	209
Breast with skin	7.6	0	29	0	193
Thigh with skin	15.4	0	24.85	0	245

Characteristics of a low-carb diet.

Elimination of wheat and other grains

- There may be a withdrawal period of a few days (about a week). Choose the timing of starting your diet carefully (avoid stressful periods).
- There is suppression of hunger because of the absence of gluten or gliadin in grains; they accelerate intestinal transit, inhibiting the production of PYY (polypeptide YY), which produces satiety.
- Lowers blood sugar to normal levels, eliminating insulin spikes.
- Other benefits include improvement in blood pressure, improvement in inflammatory processes such as eczema, seborrheic dermatitis, joint pain, and improvement of the marker of inflammation Protein C reactive.

Eat Real Food and avoid processed foods.

- Avoid any foods that come packaged in boxes, snacks, etc.
- Manage net carbohydrates to 15 g per meal, no more than 45g-50g per day.

- Fruits have large amounts of insoluble fiber, but they contain Lectin in their peel, which may produce leaky bowels, so peel them, but keep in mind the amount of sugar they contain. Beans and lentils have both soluble and insoluble fibers. Both fruits and beans are beneficial for the regularity of evacuation and slow down the absorption of sugars, avoiding the peaks and valleys of glucose in the blood and insulin levels.
- **The anti-inflammatory property** may be responsible for increased energy, better concentration, decreased joint pain, and weight loss, and may improve heartburn. (Davis, 2011)

Foods appropriate for low-car diets

Foods that satisfy and meet the nutritional requirements are easy to find; they include greens and lettuce, Asparagus, Zucchini, Tomatoes, chicken, game meats, salmon and other fish, broth, stocks, soups, and *fruits like berries.*

What diet after you have achieved your ideal weight?

Remember, you committed to a lifestyle change. You cannot go back to your pre-diet habits. It would be best to continue the newer habits you acquired while dieting: portion size, mindful eating, eating to 80% satisfaction, and stopping at that point.

Of the many different types of food preparations, the healthiest style is the Mediterranean style.

To plan a Mediterranean style of cuisine, there are a few simple points of advice:

- Add vegetables or fruit. To get enough vegetables and fruit daily, have one serving with every meal and snack.

- Choose olive oil for cooking, dressings, and as a replacement for butter in toast or bread.

- Include proteins primarily of plant origin, such as grains, beans, nuts, and meats like fish, shellfish, pork, and beef. It is probably best to limit animal proteins to once a week.

- Use herbs and spices liberally, including chilies. They add lots of flavors, minerals, and antioxidants.

Breakfasts, Side dishes and appetizers

I will first give some recipes for products that can accompany some of the main dishes or serve as appetizers.

Almond Flour Bread Inspired by **(Rider, n.d.)**

In these recipes, I would pay closer attention to the net carb content (Total carbs minus all fibers) than the caloric content. Remember that you will direct traffic away from the aerobic cycle (the significant energy producer pathway), so the dish's caloric content will not be fully utilized.

Small loaf

Ingredients for 12 servings:

Protein	Egg whites 2
	Eggs 2
Carbohydrate	Almond flour 2 cups
	Psyllium Husk powder 2 Tbsp
	Baking powder 1 ½ tsp
	Xanthan gum ½ tsp
Fat	Butter unsalted melted 2 Tbsp
Liquid	Water warm ½ cup
Seasoning	Salt ¼ tsp
Flavoring	Red onion cubed small 2 Tbsp.

Procedure:

1. Preheat the oven to 350°F and line a Bread Pan with parchment paper.
2. Beat the egg whites (4) to stiff peaks and the egg yolks to pale yellow separately. Mix ½ of the egg whites with the yolks.
3. Mix the dry ingredients in a separate bowl. Add the melted butter and water to the egg mixture.
4. Add the dry ingredients to the egg mixture and blend to a smooth dough. Now add the reserved egg whites and fold.
5. Place the batter in the prep mold and bake for 45-50 minutes. Cover the top loosely with aluminum foil if the crust is golden brown after 30 minutes.

Nutrition Total Fat 11.1g Sat. Fat 2g Total Carbs 3.4 g Fiber 1.9g Net Carbs 1.5g Calories 136

Chickpea Bread

Ingredients for 12 servings:

• Protein	Greek Yogurt 6 oz
	Eggs 4 large
	Whey protein isolates 1 cup.
	Psyllium Husk Powder 1 tbsp
• Carbohydrate	Chickpea Flour 1 cup
	Baking powder 2 tsp
	Salt ½ tsp
• Seasoning	Sesame seeds 1 Tbsp

Procedure:

1. Preheat oven to 350°F, and line one bread pan ten by 5 inches with parchment paper.
2. Mix the eggs and yogurt in a large bowl until smooth, then add all other ingredients and mix until free of lumps.

3. Bake uncovered until a toothpick comes off clean. Cover loosely with aluminum foil if the crust is golden brown before it tests done.
4. Slice when cool.
5. May freeze after slicing it.

Nutrition Total Fat 4.4g. Saturated fat 0.8g. Total-Carbs. 2.5g. Fiber 1g. Net Carbs 1.5 g. Calories 78

Chickpea Bread Turkish style Inspired by **(Kevser, 2024)**

Ingredients for 20 servings:

• Carbs	Chickpea flour 3 cups Baking soda 1 ½ tsp Stevia 1 tsp
• Liquid	Sparkling water 2 cups Vinegar white distilled or wine 1 Tbsp
• Fat	Olive oil 2 Tbsp
• Seasoning	Salt 1 tsp

Procedure:

1. Preheat the oven to 370°F.
2. In a large bowl, mix the baking soda with the vinegar until it froths. Add the sparkling water, stevia, salt, and olive oil and mix.
3. Add the chickpea flour in parts and whisk. Keep adding and whisking until the dough has a dense liquid consistency.
4. Grease a pound cake mold about 10 inches in length.
5. Bake in the oven for 40-45 minutes until a toothpick test comes out clean.

Nutrition: Total fat 3.2g. Total Carbs. 18.2g. Fiber 5.2g. Net-Carbs. 13g. Calories 121 Kcal.

Chickpea Flour Bread #2

Ingredients:

- Carbohydrates   Chickpea Flour 2 ½ cups
  - Stevia 1 ½ Tbsp
  - Baking Soda 1 ¼ tsp
- Fat   Olive oil 2Tbsp
- Liquid   Sparkling water 1 ½ cups
- Seasoning   Salt ¼ tsp

Procedure:

1. Preheat the oven to 375°F. Line a bread mold 9 x 5 inches with parchment paper.
2. Mix the flour, stevia, baking powder, and salt in a large bowl. Pour the sparkling water on the inside wall of the bowl, add the olive oil, and stir until combined.
3. Pour the batter into the prepared bread mold and bake for 40-45 minutes until the crust is golden brown and the toothpick test comes back clean.
4. Cool it before slicing (16 slices). Freeze after slicing if desired.

Nutrition Total Fat 2.7 g. Saturated fat 0.3g. Total Carbs 8.3g. Fiber 1.6g. Calories 71 Kcal.

Biscuit Recipe L.C. (low carb) inspired by (Davis MD, 2013)

Ingredients for 12 servings:

- Carbohydrates   Chickpea flour 2 cups
  - Baking Powder 1 Tbsp
- Fat   Mayonnaise ½ cup
- Seasoning   Sea Salt ½ tsp
- Liquid   Milk whole ¾ cup.

Procedure:

1. Preheat oven to 450°F
2. Mix the dry ingredients in a bowl, stirring to blend.
3. Add the mayonnaise and milk, stirring until uniform.
4. On a baking sheet lined with parchment paper, place a ¼ cup size of biscuits with enough space in between. Bake for 10 minutes or so until golden.
5. Serve it warm.

Nutrition: Total Fat 4.6 g. Saturated Fat 0.4 g. Total Carbs 16.1 g. Fiber 2.5 g. Protein 7 g. Calories 137

Chickpea Flour Taco Tortillas
inspired by (Baier, 2019)

Ingredients for sixteen servings:

- Carbohydrates   Chickpea flour 3 cups
- Liquid   Lukewarm water 3 cups
- Seasoning   Salt 1 ½ tsp
- Additions   Garlic, onions, green onions, chilis

Procedure:

1. Cook in a nonstick skillet without oil.
2. Additions of choice before butter.
3. Add batter near the center and tilt the skillet to cover the bottom.
4. When golden, flip to cook the other side.
5. Serve with the filling of your choice.

Alternatively, you may use commercially available Carb balance® or Cab Counter® tortillas.

Nutrition: Total Fat 1.2g. Saturated Fat 0.1g. Total Carbs. 10.8g. Fiber 2g. Net Carbs. 8.8g. Calories 70 kcal.

Cauliflower Fried Rice

Ingredients for four servings:

- Proteins   Eggs 2 beaten.
- Carbs   Riced Cauliflower 16 oz squeezed dry in a cheesecloth.
  Peas and carrots mix frozen 1 cup.
- Fats   Cooking spray.
  Olive oil 1 Tbsp
  Red onion small, one finely sliced.
- Aromatics   Garlic 2 cloves minced.
  Green onions, four chopped fine.
- Seasoning   Soy Sauce low sodium ¼ cup.

Procedure:

1. Heat a large skillet or a wok over medium-low heat. Spray the bottom, add the eggs, and cook an omelet when hot. Remove and set aside when ready.
2. Return the skillet to heat, add oil, and when hot, add onions; when soft, add peas and carrots. Mix and add garlic and cook for 4-5 minutes or until ready.
3. Increase the temperature to medium-high and add the dried cauliflower rice and soy sauce. Mix well and cook for about 10 minutes or until the riced cauliflower starts to sear, frequently stirring so all the cauliflower is seared about the same.
4. In the meantime, cut the omelet into small strips and add it to the skillet with the green onions at the end.
5. Serve immediately. You may add sautéed beef or chicken cut into small strips to make it a meal.

Nutrition Total Fat 4.7g. Saturated fat 0.9g. Total Carbs. 9.1g. Fiber 2.7g. Net Carbs. 6.4g.

Almost American Fried Rice

This is equivalent to the prior recipe with additional ingredients: 2 tomatoes concasse, 1 tbsp golden raisins, ham in strips, ketchup on the omelet, 1 tsp Thai fish sauce, and 1 tsp simple syrup.

Making noodles from scratch at home requires significant work; one may do this as a fan project, especially if it involves children. Otherwise, there are commercially available prepared pastas; my preference goes to two of them.

One is *Zero pasta*, produced by Nasoya® as spaghetti-shaped Shirataki or fettuccine-shaped Shirataki, produced by SKINNY and distributed by SP Global LLC., made from the root of the Konjac plant (Konnyaku. potato). It provides 4.5 to 20 calories per serving, Fats 0g, total carbohydrates 2.5 to 5g, fiber 2-3g, and Net Carbs 0-2g, depending on the choice.

The other one is produced by Kobun® and is called Healthy Noodle. It is made from soybean fiber. Each serving contains 0.5 g of fat, 6 g of total carbs, 6 g of fiber, and 0 g of net Carbs.

Both can be prepared to eat cold, warm, or stir-fried. Before boiling or stir-frying, they must be rinsed in cold water (best in a colander).

Noodles Marinara

Ingredients for two servings:

- Carbohydrates   8 oz of zero pasta or Healthy Noodles
  Red onions minced ½ cup.
- Aromatics   Tomatoes diced one can 14.5 oz or two plump tomatoes.
  Garlic minced small 1 tsp.
  Dry basil 1 tsp
- Fats   Oil canola 2 Tbsp

Procedure:

1. Heat oil in a skillet or wok.
2. Add minced onions and cook until translucent, about 2-3 minutes.
3. Add garlic and cook until fragrant.
4. Add diced tomatoes and basil and cook for about 3 minutes or until tomatoes soften.
5. Add the noodles and cook until warm.
6. Serve immediately as a side for meat or fish or as a main dish.

Nutrition: Total Fats:14.3g Sat. Fat 1.1g. Total Carbs. 10.9g. Fiber 4.7g. Net Carbs. 6.2g. Calories 170 kcal.

Pad Thai Noodles Low Carb.

Ingredients for two servings:

• Carbohydrates	8 oz of Pasta Zero® or Healthy Noodles® Bean Sprouts 1 cup
• Aromatics	Garlic minced two cloves. Green onions chopped ½ cup green and white.
• Fats	Canola oil 1 Tbsp Soy sauce 1 Tbsp Pad Thai sauce 5 Tbsp
• Seasoning and flavorings	Cilantro leaves chopped 1 Tbsp

Procedure:

1. Rinse the noodles in chilly water.
2. Heat the oil in a skillet or wok, sauté the green onions, sprouts, and garlic.
3. Add the pasta to the skillet or wok and stir fry until warm, 2 or 3 minutes.
4. Add the Pad Thai sauce, sir, to distribute evenly. Add cilantro and, if desired, lime juice of ½ a lime fruit.

5. Serve immediately as a dinner or side dish to stir-fried meat, Fish, or shellfish.

Nutrition: Total Fats 7.6g. Saturated Fats 0.5g. Total Carbs. 15.7g. Fiber 3.4g. Net Carbs. 12.3g. Calories 136 kcal.

Pizza Dough is another product we usually do not associate with home cooking. Commercially available products like cauliflower pizza dough are available. Cost may also be an issue, as the minimal size of the order would require a large amount of frozen dough that would take an inordinate amount of space in your freezer. So, I will give a simple recipe where you can control the amount made.

Cauliflower Pizza Crust Low Carb. Inspired by **(Detoximista.com, n.d.)**

Ingredients for one 11-inch Round Pie:

- Carbohydrates   Head of cauliflower one large
  Almond flour 1/2 cup
  Coconut flour ¼ cup
  Flax Powder 1 ½ tsp heaped.
- Aromatics   Ají Amarillo Paste
  Nutritional yeast 1 Tbsp

- Fats   Avocado oil 3 Tbsp
  Water 3 Tbsp
- Seasoning and flavorings   Salt and pepper to taste

Procedure:

1. Preheat oven to 450°F convection bake.
2. Remove the core and stems, add the florets to a food processor, and pulse until they become fluffy. Steam the florets for 4-5 minutes in an Asian steam basket, the bottom covered partially with parchment paper, or in a small dish.
3. Place the cauliflower rice in a cheesecloth and squeeze the excess water.

4. Whisk the water, oil, and flax powder together and knead into the cauliflower rice.
5. Add the seasonings and flour and continue kneading until the consistency is uniform. If it is too sticky, add additional flour.
6. Line a baking sheet with parchment paper, spray it with avocado oil, and press the dough into an 11-inch plate.
7. Bake at 450°F until the edges turn golden, about 18-22 minutes.
8. Remove and top the crust with your preferred ingredients. One low-carb tomato sauce available is Rao's Marinara homemade sauce, which contains 6 g of total carbohydrates, 1 g of fiber, and 5 g of net carbohydrates.

Alternatively, make a Pesto sauce using Basil leaves, toasted pine nuts, parmesan cheese, garlic, and lemon juice, and season with olive oil, salt, and pepper.

May add protein in the form of meat, chicken, or shellfish.

Nutrition: Total fat 26.5g. Saturated fat 3.2g. Total Carbs. 25.5g. Fiber 15.5g. Net Carbs 10g.

Other dishes in these groups are salads. Salads generally do not carry a heavy load of Carbohydrates unless you want a sweet dressing. Replace the sugar with stevia to keep your insulin secretion to a minimum.

I will give just examples of low-carb salads.

Spinach Salad with Roasted Fennel and Grapefruit. Inspired by (Canora, 2015)

Ingredients for six servings:

- Fennel one large bulb, halved lengthwise, then cut lengthwise ½ inch thick.
- LEAF vegetables baby spinach 5 oz
- Fruit Grapefruit pink 1.
- Olive oil 3 Tbsp
- Olives (Alfonso) cured in oil, pitted ½ cup.
- Salt and Pepper to taste

Procedure:

1. Preheat oven to 350°F. Line a baking sheet with aluminum foil.
2. Toss the fennel segments in one tablespoon of oil, season with salt and pepper, and bake until the fennel is soft and the edges are browned and crispy, about 40-45 minutes.
3. Grate the zest of the grapefruit in a bowl. Cut the top and bottom of the fruit, setting it flat and following the curvature of the grapefruit, remove the remaining skin. Cut the fruit meat between the membranes and place them in the bowl. Squeeze the remainder to place the juice in the bowl.
4. Combine the spinach, olives, and grapefruit segments in a large bowl. Save the juice for the dressing.

When the fennel is done, place it in the salad bowl with the other ingredients. Mix the juice with the remaining olive oil, taste for seasoning, and add salt and pepper.

Serve immediately.

Nutrition: Total Fat 7.3g. Saturated fat 1 g. Total Carbs. 5.3g. Fiber 2g. Net Carbs 3.3g. Calories 85g.

Grilled Radicchio with Yogurt and Toasted Hazelnuts Salad credit to **(Colender, 2015)**

Ingredients for six servings:

- Dressing
  - Olive oil 1 Tbsp
  - Onion ¾ cup finely cubed and tamed.
  - Hazelnut-infused oil (from toasting the hazelnuts)
  - Lemon Juice of ½ lemon
  - Garlic 1 clove minced.
  - Mint leaves 2 Tbsp finely chopped.
  - Yogurt whole fat plain 1 cup
  - Salt and Pepper to taste.
- For Toasted Hazelnuts
  - Raw Hazelnuts ½ cup

  - Olive oil 3 Tbsp
  - Garlic 1 clove sliced thin.
  - Thyme 1 sprig
- Salad
  - Olive oil 2 Tbsp
  - Radicchio 1 head cut into eight wedges.
  - Golden raisin ¼ cup
  - Mint leaves ¼ cup chopped finely.

Procedure:

1. Make the yogurt dressing. Sweat the onions in 1 tbsp of oil in a large skillet at medium heat until translucent; season with a 3-finger pinch of salt. Transfer to a bowl and let it cool.
2. After wiping off the hazelnut, toast it in 3 tbsp of oil in the same skillet. Cook for about 5 minutes, stirring frequently until toasted. Add the sliced garlic and the thyme sprig and cook until fragrant, a few additional seconds. Reserve the hazelnut-infused oil.
3. Once the onions are excellent, fold the yogurt, lemon juice, and minced garlic—strain 2 tbsp of the infused oil.
4. Grill the radicchio wedges on medium-high heat after tossing them in a bowl with olive oil, salt, and pepper. Grill until the edges are slightly charred, turn over, and cook until cooked through, for about 3-4 minutes.
5. Serve the salad with the grilled wedges in the center of the plate. Spoon over the dressing, top with the dressing, and garnish with raisins and mint leaves.

Nutrition Total Fat 15.8 g. Saturated fat2.5g. Total Carbs. 9.8g. fiber 1.5g. Net Carbs. 8.3 Calories 184 Kcal.

Grilled Cesar Cabbage Salad (Carmellini, 2017)

Ingredients for four servings:

• Green leafy Vegetable	Green Cabbage quartered 1
• Fats	Olive oil ¼ cup
	Parmesan cheese grated 2 Tbsp.
• Protein	Anchovy fillets minced 2 tsp
• Carbs.	Capers minced 2 tsp
	Wasa Crisp Bread 2 slices for garnish as crumbs
• Seasoning and Flavoring	Salt and Pepper to taste
	Ají Amarillo 1 tsp
• Fruits	Orange juice 2 Tbsp
	Raisins golden 1 Tbsp
	Orange zest 1 tsp

Procedure:

1. Grill the quartered Cabbage on a hot grill until well charred on all sides, for about 7 minutes per side. Transfer the cabbage to a bowl and cover it with plastic wrap to steam for 15 minutes.
2. In a small bowl, whisk the olive oil, orange juice, raisins, minced anchovies, capers, garlic, orange zest, chili paste, salt, and pepper.
3. Remove the core of the cabbage and cut the leaves into 1-inch pieces, then toss with the dressing. Transfer to a platter and garnish with a fillet of anchovy, grated cheese, and Wasa crispy breadcrumbs.

Nutrition Total Fats 17.1 g. Saturated Fats 3.4g. Total Carbs. 22.8g. Fiber 5.6g. Net Carbs. 17.3g Calories 271 kcal.

Another group of dishes that fit this category is soups, which I will give examples of now.

Celeriac Leek Cream Soup Inspired by **(Fearnley-Whittingstall, 1999)**

Ingredients for ten servings:

Makes 1.4 lt. or 2 ½ pt.

• Protein	Bacon 6 slices
• Carbohydrate	Celeriac peeled and cubed 20 oz
• Fat	Oil canola 1 1/3 Tbsp
	Butter unsalted or Ghee1 Tbsp
	Heavy cream 3 ½ fluid oz
• Aromatics	Red Onion finely sliced.
	Leeks sliced in half, cleaned and sliced.
	Garlic 2 cloves pressed.
• Seasonings and flavorings	Sea salt and freshly ground black pepper are used to taste.
	Bay leaves 2
	Cilantro chopped 2 Tbsp.
• Liquid	Vegetable stock 4 cups

Procedure:

1. Heat the oil and butter in a heavy stock pot. When shimmering, add the onion, leeks, and bay leaf. Turn the heat down to medium-low and sweat them for 10 minutes. Add the celeriac and sweat it for another 5 minutes. Add the vegetable stock and simmer until the celeriac starts breaking down.
2. While simmering, cook the bacon, turning it over, until crispy. Drain it on a paper towel.
3. When the soup is ready, remove it from the heat, add the cream, and blend with a submersion blender until smooth. Serve in little cups and sprinkle with bacon pieces and cilantro.

Nutrition: Total Fat 11.7g. Saturated Fat 4.9g. Total Carbohydrates 10.1g. Fiber 1.8g. Net Carbs. 8.3g.

Tomato Aspic inspired by **(Southern living test Kitchen , 2024)**

Ingredients for four servings:

- Protein   Gelatin 0.25 oz unflavored
- Aromatics   Onions ½ cup cubed small.
  Celery ½ cup cubed small peeled.
- Liquid   Boiling water ¼ cup
  Vegetable Juice 2 cups (V8?)
- Flavorings   Bay Leaf 1
  Cloves 2
  Worcestershire sauce one dash

Procedure:

1. Dissolve gelatin in the boiling water and set aside.
2. Combine vegetable juice, Worcestershire sauce, bay leaf, and cloves in a saucepan and bring to a boil. Reduce heat and simmer for 10 minutes or so to infuse the liquid. Discard the bay leaf and the cloves.
3. Stir onions and celery into vegetable juice, pour the mixture over the gelatin solution, and stir to mix.
4. Pour in serving plates and refrigerate until set completely.

Nutrition Total Fat 0.1g. Saturated Fat 0g. Total Carbs 7.5g. Fiber 1.7g. Net Carbs 5.8g. Calories 42

Oven Roasted Tomatoes (Keller, 2012)

Ingredients for eight tomatoes halves:

- Vegetables   Plum tomatoes 4
- Fats   Olive oil 2 Tbsp
- Flavoring   Thyme leaves, chopped 1 tsp
- Seasoning   Salt and Pepper to taste

Procedure

1. Preheat oven to 275°F. Fill a bowl with ice water. Fill a stock pot with water and boil it.
2. Prepare the tomatoes by marking an X at the bottom and existing shallowing the stem. Place the tomatoes in boiling water for about 30 seconds; the skin should loosen up. Set them in the ice water to stop the cooking. Carefully peel the skin.
3. Place the tomatoes in a non-stick baking pan, drizzle with olive oil, add the thyme leaves, and season with salt and pepper.
4. Roast the tomatoes until tender and slightly shrunken, about 2 ½ hours. Transfer the tomatoes to a plate and set aside to cool.

Nutrition Total fat 3.6g. Saturated Fat 0.5g. Total Carbs. 2.5g. Fiber 0.8g. Net Carbs. 1.7g. Calories 41

Scallops Appetizer with Mustard Mayonnaise inspired by (Lagasse, n.d.)

Ingredients: for six servings

- Protein   Egg Yolks 4 large
- Seasoning   Mustard Dijon 1Tbsp
                     Ají amarillo paste 2 tsp
                     Salt and Pepper to taste
                     Vinegar, warm 2 Tbsp
- Fats   Olive oil 2 Tbsp

<table>
<tr><td>• Flavoring agents</td><td>Canola oil ½ cup
Worcestershire sauce 1 tsp
Tomato paste 1 ½ Tbsp
Cilantro leaves chopped 1 tsp.
Thyme leaves 1 tsp
Oregano leaves chopped 1 tsp.</td></tr>
<tr><td>• Side dish</td><td>Asparagus 18 stalks</td></tr>
</table>

Procedure:

1. Prepare the mayonnaise by placing an immersion blender in a container that will allow it to reach the bottom. Place the ingredients in the order listed. Run the immersion blender slowly from the bottom upward as the mayo thickens to the desired consistency.
2. Boil the asparagus until al dente. Place it in a bowl with iced water for 10 minutes.
3. Place a lettuce leaf on each plate to serve the scallops.
4. Sear the scallops in a hot skillet with some oil. Sear the presentation side first for a couple of minutes; do not turn until they are golden brown and not adherent to the bottom. Flip them over and repeat the searing. Do not overcook them, or they will become tough.
5. Serve over the lettuce leaf, asparagus on the side, and a dollop of spicy mayonnaise.

Nutrition: Total Fat 26.3g. Saturated fat 3.2g. Total Carbs. 5.5g. Fiber 1.5g. Net Carbs. 4g. Calories 300

Olive and Caper Spread

Ingredients for 20 servings:

- Roast a bulb of garlic at 375°F for 1 hour.
- Roast 3 to 4 slices of lemon for 45 minutes.
- Roast Cappers 2 Tbsp
- green olives 1 cup,
- Roast ½ ich thick slice of Onion for 50 minutes

- Carb — Maple syrup 3 Tbs.
  Lemon marmalade 1 ½ Tbsp
- Aromatics — One clove
- Nuts — ¼ cup pistachios soaked to soften.
  Cashews ¼ cup soaked.
- Fats — Olive oil 1/3 cup
- Liquids — Water ½ cup
  White wine 3 Tbsp
- Flavoring — Ají Amarillo ½ teaspoon ground

Procedure

1. Cool all roasted ingredients before blending.
2. Put all ingredients in a blender and blend for 1 minute.
3. Add chopped coriander and season to taste.
4. Chill in the refrigerator to thicken.
5. May serve with Wasa crispy bread segments of appropriate size.

Nutrition: Total fat 2.3g. Sat. Fat 0.1g. Total Carbs 9.4g. Fiber 0.9g. Net Carbs 8.5g. Calories 59

Tuna Sashimi with Fennel Apple Salad

Ingredients for four servings:

Tuna
- 8 oz sushi-grade tuna
- 1/2 cup pickled ginger julienned Avocado

Puree
- one ripe avocado
- 2 tbsp lemon juice
- salt

Vinaigrette
- 1 tbsp ají paste
- 1/4 cup orange juice
- salt

Ponzu
- 1/2 cup soy sauce
- 1 tsp ginger, peeled and
- 2-3 tbsp lemon juice

Salad
- one fennel bulb
- one fuji apple
- 2cups mesclun salad mix

Garnish
- Vietnamese rice paper rolls, broiled until crispy, 15–30 seconds
- radish slices
- fennel pollen
- Fresno chili pepper slices
- red jalapeño slices
- edible flowers or bean sprouts

Procedure

1. Start with the avocado puree. Cut the avocado into quarters. Remove the pit and scrape out the contents with a spoon. Pass it through a tamis or blend it in a small food processor. Squeeze in the lemon juice and season with salt. Taste.
2. Next, make the vinaigrette. Combine the chili paste and orange juice in a small bowl. Stir well—season with salt and set aside.
3. Move on to the ponzu sauce. In another small bowl, add the soy sauce. Grate in ginger using a Microplane. Squeeze in lemon juice. mix and taste. Dilute to taste with a broth of your choice.
4. To make the salad, slice the fennel bulb and the apple on a mandolin. Then, julienne the slices and place them in a small bowl. Cut the mesclun greens and add them to the apple and fennel. Season the salad with salt.
5. Immediately dress with the ají chili vinaigrette to prevent the apples from browning. Taste.
6. Now cut the tuna on an angle into pieces about ⅛ an inch thick. Put ½ tsp ginger on each slice of tuna and roll up.

Nutrition: Total fat 9.7g. Saturated fat1.4g. Total Carbs 27.9g. Fiber 7.8g. Net Carbs 20.1g. Calories 258 kcal.

Brussels Sprouts and Bacon

Ingredients for eight servings:

- Protein   Bacon 4 slices chopped.
- Carbohydrates   Brussel Sprouts washed and halved 1.5 lb.
- Fats   Olive oil 2 Tbsp
- Seasonings   Salt ½ tsp
         Black Pepper ¼ tsp
- Flavoring   Balsamic vinegar 4 oz

Procedure:

1. Preheat the oven to 425°F.
2. Toss the Brussels sprouts in a bowl with olive oil. Place them on a baking sheet and season with salt and Pepper.
3. Add chopped bacon to the baking sheet and roast them for 20-25 minutes. Flip the Brussels sprouts at mid-point. They are done when lightly browned.
4. In the meantime, reduce the balsamic vinegar to the point that it is thickened.
5. When the Brussels sprouts are done, remove them from the oven and drizzle the balsamic reduction over them.

Nutrition Total Fat 7.8g. Saturated Fat 1.9g. Total Carbohydrates 10.6g. Fiber 3.3g. Net Carbs. 7.3g. Calories 129

Main Dishes Low Carbohydrates for Weight Loss

Beef recipes.

Anticuchos of Beef Heart

Ingredients for four servings: (2 sticks per serving)

- Protein   One beef heart or beef tenderloin 2 lbs.

For the Marinade:

- Aromatics   Garlic 5 cloves pressed.
- Spices   Cumin ½ Tbsp
  Ají Panca ½ cup.
- Herbs   Oregano ground 2 tsp
- Seasonings   Salt and pepper to taste
- Liquid   Vinegar¾ cup
- Fat   Canola oil 1½ cups
- To accompany   Sweet Potatoes and Corn on the cob

Procedure:

1. Clean the heart, removing the fat, membranes, valves, and large blood vessels. Leave only the meat.
2. Cut the meat transversely and at a slight angle into pieces, about an inch and a quarter.
3. Mix the aromatics, spices, seasonings, oregano, and liquid in a large bowl.
4. Marinate the heart pieces in the mixture from #3 for at least 2 hours, best overnight.
5. Place about 3 or 4 pieces of heart in a shish kebab stick. I often use two sticks parallel in the meat so that when you turn them, the meat will not slide around.
6. Grill in a very hot grill. Baste them with the marinade every so often.
7. Serve them with a piece of corn on the cob, pieces of boiled potatoes, and an ají sauce, either rocoto (hotter) or amarillo.

Nutrition Total fat 9.2g. Saturated fat 3.2g. Total Carbohydrates 0g. Protein 24.6 g. Calories 190Kcal.

Beef Burgundy with Noodles inspired by **(Taste of Home, 2023)**

Ingredients for two servings:

• Protein	Beef top sirloin steak cut into ¼ inch strips. Mushrooms quartered 1 ½ cup.
• Carbs.	Shirataki noodles Pasta Zero 2 cups Potatoes flour 2 tsp
• Fats	Butter, unsalted 2 tsp Beef demiglace or Better than Bouillon beef base ½ tsp
• Seasoning and flavoring	Sea Salt or Kosher ¼ tsp Black Pepper freshly ground 1/8 tsp. Fresh Parsley minced 3 Tbsp divided. Bay Leaf 1 Clove 1 whole Onion red medium, cubed medium.

| | Scallions 4 stalks segmented in ¼ -inch segments. |
| • Liquid | Wine red ¾ cup
Water 1/3 cup, divided. |

Procedure

1. Heat the butter in a Dutch oven. When melted and shimmering, add the beef and onions, and sauté until the meat is golden brown. Add the mushrooms, wine, ¼ cups of water, 2 Tbs. of parsley, and seasonings. Bring to a boil. Reduce the heat to simmering, cover, and simmer until the beef is tender, about 1 hour.
2. In a nonstick skillet, stir the Pasta zero fettuccini with cooking spray until lightly browned. Time this step to be ready when the beef stew is ready. Add the segmented scallions towards the end.
3. If desired, add the demiglace or Bullion to intensify the beef flavor of the sauce.
4. After discarding the bay leaf and the clove, use the remaining flour to prepare a slurry to thicken the sauce of the beef mixture.
5. Serve over the noodles and sprinkle with remaining parsley.

Nutrition Total Fat 10g. Sat. Fat 5g. Total Carbs. 7.9g. Fiber 3.7g. Net Carbs. 4.2g. Calories 338

Stir fry of Beef and Broccoli.

Ingredients for two servings:

• Protein	Beef Top Sirloin Steak ½ lb. cut into ¼ inch thick strips
• Carbs	Stevia 1 Tbsp Cornstarch 1 Tbsp
• Fat	Canola oil 2 tsp divided.
• Vegetables	Broccoli florets 2 cups.
• Aromatics	Garlic 1 clove minced. Gingerroot minced small 1 tsp Green onions eight stalks cut into 1-inch pieces.

- Liquid   Beef broth reduced sodium ½ cup.
  Sherry ¼ cup
  Soy sauce reduced sodium 2 Tbsp.

Procedure

1. Heat 1 tsp of oil in a large nonstick skillet and stir fry the beef strips until browned, about 2-3 minutes. Remove from the pan.
2. Stir fry the broccoli in the second teaspoon of oil until crisp and tender, 1-2 minutes. Add the green onions and cook until tender, 1-2 minutes.
3. Mix all remaining ingredients in a bowl, add them to the skillet, stir, and cook until thickened.
4. Add the beef and warm through.
5. May serve with cauliflower rice or low-carb noodles.

Nutrition Total fat 12.7 g. Saturated fat 3.4g. Total Carbs. 11.8g. Fiber 0.2g. Net Carbs. 11.6 Calories 305Kcal.

Beef Wonton Empanadas

Ingredients for 18 Empanadas:

- Protein   Ground beef 1 lb.
  Eggs 1 large
- Carbs.   Wonton wrappers.
- Fat   Oil Canola 1 Tbsp
  Mexican Blend shredded cheese
- Aromatics   Onions diced 1 cup.
  Red Bell Pepper diced ½ cup.
  Tomato paste ¼ cup.
- Seasoning and flavorings   Sea Salt 1 tsp
  Black Pepper ¾ tsp
  Cumin 2 tsp
  Paprika 1 tsp
  Capers chopped 2Tbsp
  Parsley chopped ¼ cup.
- Liquid   lime Juice of 2 limes

Procedure:

1. Preheat oven to 400°F. Heat a heavy skillet; when hot, add oil; when shimmering, it may begin to cook.
2. Add diced onion and sauté until translucent, about 5 minutes. Then add diced Bell Pepper and cook for another 5 minutes. Add ground beef and brown it through.
3. Turn the heat off and add the capers and parsley. Let it cool, then add lime juice.
4. Set up a station to assemble the empanadas. Make an egg wash (1 egg and 1 Tbsp water). From left to right, position the beef mixture, cheese, wonton wrappers, small bowl with water, space to work, and a baking sheet and the egg wash bowl to the right of this workspace.
5. Place one wonton wrapper on your work area surface. Put 2 tsp of beef mixture in the lower 1/3 of the wrapper. Sprinkle the shredded cheese on the beef, fold the wrapper, wet the edges with water, and seal from the center to the corners, pushing toward the edge.
6. Place the empanada on the baking sheet and brush with the egg wash. Roast for 15 minutes in a 400°F oven.
7. Serve while still warm.

Nutrition Total fat 7g. Sat. Fat 2g. Total Carbs. 5 g. Fiber 1g. Net Carbs. 4g. Calories 112 Kcal.

Beef Fajitas

Ingredients for eight servings:

• Protein	Beef skirt steak 1 ½ lb. in strips.
• Carbs.	Chickpea Tortillas Chickpea Flour **Taco** Tortillas inspired by *Chickpea Flour Taco Tortillas* ***inspired*** *by* Sweet onion large one sliced thick Red Bell Pepper 4 sliced and seeded. Cooking Spray
Fat	Grated Lime Zest 1 tsp

- • Seasonings and Flavorings — Garlic 4 cloves

  Ají Amarillo ground 1 tsp
  Sea Salt ¾ tsp
  Black Pepper ¾ tsp
  Ají Amarillo paste 2 tsp
  ½ cup Tequila or low-sodium beef broth
- • Liquid — ½ cup of lime juice

Procedure:

1. Mix the liquids, seasonings, and flavorings in a bowl. Divide into two bowls.
2. Add peppers and onion to one bowl.
3. Cut the skirt steaks in half and add to the second bowl.
4. Cover both with plastic wrap and refrigerate for several hours or overnight.
5. Drain beef and vegetables. Discard marinade.
6. In a preheated grill or a grilling pan with cooking spray, grill the onions and peppers until crisp-tender. You may add a squirt of vinegar at the end. Simultaneously, in a different pan, cook the skirt steaks to the preferred temperature of 125-135°F for medium rare and 160°F for medium. Let them rest for 5 minutes.
7. Serve in the chickpea tortillas and top with cheese.

Nutrition Total fat 11.7g. Saturated fat 5.4g. Total Carbs. 15.5g. Fiber 2g. Net Carb.13.5g.

Calories 241Kcal.

Beef and Mushrooms Stuffed Zucchini Boats

Ingredients for 8servings:

- • Protein — Lean ground beef 1 lb.
- • Fat — Cheddar cheese shredded ½ cup

- Carb
- Aromatics   Onion large diced small 1
  Red Bell Pepper diced small 1.
  Tomato sauce 1 ½ cups
  Salsa ½ cup
- Vegetable   Zucchini medium 4
  Mushrooms shitake 8 0z.
- Seasoning   Pepper ¼ tsp
  Salt ¼ tsp

Procedure

1. Preheat the oven to 350°F. Cut each zucchini lengthwise, scooping out the flesh, leaving a ¼ "shell. Chop the flesh and set aside.
2. In a large skillet, cook the beef, onion, red bell pepper, and mushrooms until the meat is no longer pink, breaking it into crumbles.
3. Stir in tomato sauce, black pepper, and zucchini flesh. Bring to a boil, reduce heat, and simmer uncovered for 10 minutes.
4. Stir in salsa and spoon the mixture into the zucchini shells. Place them in a baking dish coated with cooking spray.
5. Bake covered for about 20 minutes, sprinkle with cheese, and bake uncovered until zucchini is tender and filling is heated through.

Nutrition Total Fat 15.7g. Saturated Fat 7.2g. Total Carbs. 16.8g. Fiber 3.8g. Net Carbs. 13g. Calories 326 kcal.

Beef in Lettuce Wraps with an Orange Touch.

Ingredients for eight servings:

For the stuffing

- Protein   1 ½ lb. lean ground beef (90% lean)
- Carbs.   Stevia 1 Tbsp
  Orange marmalade 1 Tbsp
  Cornstarch 2 tsp

- Leafy Vegetables   Shredded carrots 1 cup.
          Cauliflower rice fried 2 cups.
          Boston Lettuce leaves 8.
- Aromatics   Garlic 2 cloves minced.
          Ginger root minced 2 tsp
          Green onions, three stalks thinly sliced.
- Liquid   Soy sauce reduced sodium ¼ cup.
          Orange juice 2 Tbsp
          Water ¼ cup
- Seasonings and Flavorings Ají Amarillo powder 1 tsp
- Fat   Cooking spray canola oil.

Procedure:

1. In a small bowl, mix the sauce ingredients.
2. Spray a large nonstick skillet with canola oil and cook the beef over medium-high heat to brown it, stirring to crumble the meat. Drain any residual liquid. Stir in soy sauce, orange marmalade, and ají amarillo powder. Prepare a slurry with corn starch and water and stir it into the pan a bit at a time when it does not thicken anymore.
3. Serve over lettuce leaves with fried cauliflower (see side dishes and appetizers), cover with beef mixture, and top with carrots and green onions.

Nutrition: Total fat 8.8g. Sat. Fat 3.4g. Total Carbs. 15.2g. Fiber 0.7g. Net Carbs. 14.5g. Calories 226 Kcal.

Ropa Vieja (Pulled Beef)

Ingredients for eight servings:

- Protein   Chuck Roast Beef 3 lb.
- Carbohydrates   Bell Red Pepper seeded and thinly sliced.

	Green Bell Pepper seeded and thinly sliced.
• Fats	Cooking Spray
• Aromatics	Onion 1 Medium thinly sliced.
	Garlic 3 cloves minced or compressed.
	Tomatoes crushed 14 oz can.
• Seasoning and Flavoring	Salt 2 tsp
	Black Pepper 1 tsp
	Cumin 1 Tbsp
	Pimenton 2 tsp
	Oregano 2 tsp
	Allspice ¼ tsp
	Cloves ¼ tsp
• Liquids	Beef Broth 2 cups
	Juice of 1 lime
• Chickpea tortillas	8 Chickpea Flour Taco Tortillas inspired by *Chickpea Flour* Taco Tortillas **inspired** by

Procedure:

1. Mix all the seasoning, flavorings, and garlic in a small bowl.
2. Prepare the mushrooms by simmering them in one cup of beef broth with one cup of beef demi glace or one tsp of better-than-bouillon beef base.
3. Sauté the sliced peppers and onions in a nonstick skillet until translucent. Mix with the mushroom preparation and then the second cup of beef broth (Braising liquid).
4. Rub the spice mixture over the chuck roast, place it in a saucepan, add the Braising liquid, and simmer until the roast's internal temperature is about 125°F. Then turn the heat off, remove the saucepan from the hot burner, and rest for 5-10 minutes, checking the roast's internal temperature, which should be no higher than 135- 140°F. Uncover, shred, and serve with the mushrooms and vegetables in a chickpea tortilla.

Nutrition Total fat 47.8 g. Saturated fat 19g. Total carbs 5g. Fiber 1.1g Net 3.9g. Calories 646 Kcal. Remember to add the nutrition data of the chickpea tortillas.

Beef Top Round Roast with an Italian Flair

Ingredients for eight servings:

- Protein   Beef Top Round Steak 3-5 lb.
- Carbs   Tomato sauce 8 oz
                          Corn starch 1 Tbsp
- Fat   Canola oil 2Tbsap.
- Aromatics   Onion Soup mix 2 Tbsp
                          Garlic 3 cloves sliced 1/16 inch thick.
- Liquid   Red wine vinegar 2 Tbsp
                          Water 1 Tbsp
                          ¼ cup of beef broth
- Seasonings and flavorings   Pepper ¼ tsp
                          Oregano 1tsp of leaves

Procedure:

1. Preheat the oven to 325°F. Prepare the roast by stabbing it multiple times with a paring knife and inserting garlic slices in each. Mix 1 tbsp of the oil with 1 tsp of cumin, the oregano, and the onion soup mix. Brush this mixture on all sides of the roast.
2. Roast the meat for 1 ½ hours (for a four lb. roast), internal temperature 130°F, and rest for 15-20 minutes.
3. Mix the vinegar, broth, 1 tsp of beef base better than bouillon, pepper, and mushrooms. At the appropriate time, cook the mushrooms in this mix for the sauce.
4. May be accompanied with cauliflower fried rice, scalloped potatoes, and asparagus.
5. Cut across the grain in ½ inch-thick slices.

Nutrition Total fat 16g. Sat. Fat 8g. Total Carbs. 4.7g. Fiber 0.8g. Calories 325 Kcal.

Beef Lo Mein with Spinach

Ingredients for five servings:

- Protein — Top Round steak thinly sliced 1 lb.
- Carbohydrates — Pasta Zero Shirataki spaghetti three packages.
  Water Chestnuts sliced one can.
- Fats — Sesame oil 2 tsp
  Canola oil 4 tsp
- Aromatics — Garlic cloves diced.
  Green onions, two stalks sliced ½ inch thick.
- Leafy vegetable — Baby spinach 10 oz Package coarsely chopped.
- Liquid — Water 1 Tbsp
- Flavorings — Hoisin sauce ¼ cup
  Soy sauce 2 Tbsp
  Ají Amarillo powder ¼ tsp
  Ají Amarillo paste 2 tsp

Procedure:

1. Mix hoisin sauce, soy sauce, water, sesame seed oil, garlic, and ají Amarillo powder in a small bowl. Remove ¼ cups of the mix and place it in a large bowl. Add the beef and marinate for one-quarter hour.
2. Sauté the Pasta Zero with cooking spray until slightly toasted. Set aside.
3. Heat 2 tsp of canola oil in a large skillet. Increase heat to medium-high, add ½ the beef mixture and 15 oz tomato sauce, and stir fry until no longer pink. Set aside.
4. Add the remaining canola oil and stir fry the water chestnuts, green onion, and ají amarillo paste for ½ minutes. Stir in the spinach and the remainder of the hoisin mixture that was set aside initially. Cook until the spinach is done.
5. Add Pasta zero, stir to combine, and heat through.
6. Serve the combination on a flat plate.

Nutrition Total fat 14.5g. Sat. Fat 3.9g. Total Carbs. 9.8g. Fiber 3.5g. Net Carbs 6.3g Calories 293 kcal.

Beef Bake Low Carbs

Ingredients for eight servings:

- Protein   Ground beef lean 1.5 lb.
- Carbs   Cauliflower rice 12 oz
- Fats   Sour cream ½ cup

    Cottage cheese one ¼ cup

    Two cups shredded Cheddar cheese.

- Aromatics   Tomato sauce 15 oz can

    Green onions slice (1/2 inch) ½ cup

- Seasoning   Sea Salt 1 tsp

    Black Pepper 1 tsp

Procedure:

1. Preheat oven to 350°F.
2. Because cauliflower rice contains a significant amount of water, it is best to place it in a cheesecloth and, using hand pressure, remove as much water as possible before cooking. Then, in a skillet, toast or stir-fry the cauliflower rice.
3. Then place the toasted cauliflower rice at the bottom of a casserole dish 8x8 inch.
4. In a sauce pot, cook the beef in cooking spray until browned, stirring often to crumble it. Drain the excess juice/water, then add the tomato sauce, salt, and pepper. Set Aside.
5. In a mixing bowl, stir the cottage cheese and sour cream, and mix the green onions.
6. Mix ½ of the cream-cottage cheese over the cauliflower rice in the casserole dish—layer half of the ground beef mixture and top with ½ of the cheddar cheese. Repeat a second layer of cream-cottage cheese and beef mixture and finish with the shredded cheddar cheese.
7. Bake at the pre-heated temperature for 20-25 minutes. Broil for a minute or two to brown the surface cheese.

Nutrition Total fat 23.9g. Sat. Fat 12g. Total Carbs 9g. Fiber 2g. Net Carbs 7g Calories 380 kcal.

Chickpea Tortilla Casserole

Ingredients for four servings:

- Protein Ground beef lean (90%) ½ lb.
- Carbs *4* Chickpea Flour Taco Tortillas inspired by
  Chickpea Flour Taco Tortillas **inspired** by
- Fats Ricotta Cheese ¾ cup
  Mozzarella cheese shredded ¼ cup.
  Cheddar cheese shredded ½ cup.
- Aromatics Onion chopped ½ cup
  Garlic minced two cloves.
  Tomatoes canned diced canned 14 ½ oz
- Flavorings Ají Amarillo powder 1 tsp
  Cumin ground ½ tsp
  Cilantro fresh leaves minced 3 tbsp

Procedure:

1. Preheat oven to 400°F
2. In a large skillet, crumble ground beef with onions and garlic until no longer pink, about 4-5 minutes. Stir in flavoring and tomatoes with the juices. Bring to a boil; remove from the heat.
3. Mix ricotta cheese, mozzarella, and 2 tbsp of cilantro leaves in a small bowl.
4. Place a tortilla in a baking recipient coated with cooking spray, where it can lay flat. Layer with ½ of the beef mixture, another tortilla, the ricotta mixture, another tortilla, and the remaining meat sauce. Top with the remaining tortilla and sprinkle with cheddar cheese and cilantro.
5. Bake until heated through, about 15 to 20 minutes.

Nutrition Total fat 12.4g. Saturated fat 6.7g. Total Carbs 15.8g. Fiber 1.4g. Net Carbs 14.4g. Calories 22 kcal.

Chicken Dishes

Chicken with Artichokes Casserole.

Ingredients for eight servings:

- Protein   Eight boneless skinless chicken breast halves (about 4oz)
  Mushrooms, preferably shitake 4-5 oz
- Carbohydrates   Chickpea flour 1/3 cup
  Noodles Pasta zero shirataki ® or Healthy Noodle sautéed.
  Artichokes quartered canned 8 oz
- Fat   Butter 2 Tbsp
- Seasonings   Sea Salt and Black pepper to taste
- Flavorings   Rosemary dry 1 ½ tsp
  Parsley fresh minced 1 Tbsp
- Aromatics   Red Onion chopped ½ cup.
- Liquid   Chicken broth 2 cups low sodium

Procedure:

1. Preheat the oven to 350°F
2. Browning the protein. In a large nonstick skillet, brown the chicken breasts until crispy and tender.
3. Transfer the browned chicken breasts to a 13x8.5-inch Baking dish. Arrange them with some space between them. Arrange the mushrooms and artichokes on top of the chicken.
4. Sauté the onions in the pan juices from browning the chicken. Add the salt, pepper, and chickpea flour, stirring until blended. Add the chicken broth, boil, and cook until thickened. Pour over the chicken preparation into the baking dish.
5. Bake uncovered until the internal temperature of the chicken reaches 165°F (40-45 minutes)
6. Serve with noodles and sprinkle with parsley leaves.

Note: I prefer canned artichokes because marinated ones have a bit of a bitter taste.

Nutrition Total fat 7.2. Saturated fat 1.9. Total Carbs 6.6g. Fiber 2.6g. Net Carbs. 4g. Calories 235 kcal.

Chicken Thighs Braised with Apples and Onion. Inspired by (Hammer, 2021)

Ingredients for four servings:

- Protein   Chicken thighs with skin and bone in
- Carbohydrates   Apples 2 Gala or Fuji or Honey crisp
                   Stevia 2 tbsp diluted in 3 tbsp of water.
- Fats   Canola oil 1 Tbsp
- Aromatics   Red Onion 1 medium sliced medium thickness
                   Garlic 1-2 cloves pressed.
- Seasonings   Sea Salt 3 Three-finger sprinkles (1/4 tsp)
                   Black pepper, freshly ground, two three-finger sprinkles.
- Flavorings   BBQ sugar-free sauce like G Hughes Smokehouse® or
                   Primal Kitchen BBQ Sauce 1/3 cup.
                   Apple cider or juice ¼ cup.

Procedure

1. Heat the oil, brown the chicken thighs in a large nonstick skillet, and make the skin golden brown. I often tie the thigh into a cylinder, covering the meat with the skin. Set aside in a baking dish, add the chopped apples in medium cubes, and cover with aluminum foil.

2. Add sliced onion to the pan and cook until transparent at medium heat. Add the garlic and cook for a minute or so. Stir the BBQ sauce and cider to recover the fond from browning the chicken

3. Pour over the chicken and apples and Bake in a preheated oven to 400°F, to the chicken's internal temperature of 165°F, for about 13-15 minutes at 400°F.

4. Serve the chicken with apples and onions. It may accompany either cauliflower sauté rice or pasta Zero sauté noodles.

Nutrition: Total fat 19.5g. Saturated fat 4.8g. Total Carbs 21.4g. Fiber 2.7g. Net Carbs 18.7g. Calories

Chicken Burrito Skillet

Ingredients for six servings:

- Protein   Chicken breasts skinless boneless one lb. cut in 1 ½ "
- Aromatics   Onion powder ½ tsp
  Garlic powder ½ tsp
  Ají Amarillo powder ½ tsp
  Tomatoes diced can of 14 ½ oz 1 can.
  Tomato medium chopped.
  Green onions chopped 3.
- Fat   Olive Oil 2 Tbsp
  Mexican cheese mix shredded 1 cup.
- Flavorings   Cumin ground 1 tsp
- Liquid   Chicken broth without salt 2 ½ cup
- Other   Black Bean 1 can 15oz rinsed and drained
- Cauliflower rice   1 ½ cup

Procedure:

1. Toss chicken with salt and pepper. In a large cast iron skillet, heat 1 Tbsp of oil over medium-high heat until shimmering. Sauté chicken until browned (about 2 minutes). Remove from pan and set aside.
2. In the same pan, heat the remaining oil over medium-high heat, sauté rice until lightly browned, then remove from the pan and set aside. Stir in beans, canned tomatoes, seasoning and flavorings, and broth. Bring to a boil. Place chicken on top, not pushing it into the beans, and simmer until it is no longer pink, about 20-25 minutes. Add then the toasted cauliflower rice.
3. Remove from heat and sprinkle with cheese. Let stand covered until the cheese is melted. Top with chopped tomatoes and green onions.

Nutrition: Total fat 18.7g. Saturated Fat 7.4g. Total Carbs 23.1g. Fiber 10.3g. Net Carbs 12.8g. Calories 375 kcal.

Chicken (Sautéed) with Coconut Milk

Ingredients for four servings:

- Protein — Four skinless, boneless chicken breast halves
- Aromatics — One red onion chopped.
  Fresh ginger 1 Tbsp
  Garlic 2 cloves minced.
  Three tomatoes in concasse (peeled and seeded tomatoes)
- Spices — Ground cumin 1 tsp
  Ají Amarillo ground 1 tsp
  Turmeric 1 tsp
  Ground coriander seeds.
- Herbs — Cilantro 1 bunch
- Seasonings — Salt and pepper
- Liquid — Coconut milk light 14 oz
- Fat — 2 Tbsp of vegetable oil

Procedure:

1. mix all the aromatics and spices except the tomatoes in a medium bowl. Add Salt and Pepper to taste. Place the chicken in the bowl and brush all sides with the spice mixture.

2. Heat the pan, then add one tablespoon of vegetable oil and heat it until shimmering. Sauteed the chicken 75% show side down, then turned over and cooked the other side. Remove and rest on a plate.

3. Add the remaining 1 Tbsp of oil to the same pan. Cook the aromatics and spices from the bowl except the tomatoes for a few minutes, then add the tomatoes and continue to cook for 5 minutes. Add the coconut milk cold (to deglaze the pan) and heat it. Bring the chicken back to the pan and reheat. Pour the sauce over the chicken to serve.

Nutrients: Total fat 15g. Saturated fat 9.5g. Total Carbs 8.4g. Fiber 1.5g. Net Carbs 6.9g. Calories 276

Chicken Fajitas

Ingredients for six servings:

- Protein   Chicken breasts boneless, skinless 1 ½ lb. cut into strips
- Carbohydrates   Bell Pepper red ½ julienned.
  Bell Pepper green julienned
  Six chickpea flour tortillas or Carb counter tortillas are commercially available.
- Fats   Canola oil 6 Tbsp divided.
- Aromatics   Red onion sliced medium thickness ½ cup.
  Green onions, sliced ¼ inch four.
  Garlic 3 cloves pressed.
- Seasoning   Sea Salt and Black pepper to taste
- Flavorings   Oregano dry 1 ½ tsp or double fresh
  Cumin ground 1 ½ tsp
  Ají Amarillo powder 1 tsp
  Pimenton or smoked Paprika ½ tsp
- Liquid   Lime juice 2 Tbsp
- Toppings   Choose from Shredded cheddar cheese, pico de gallo, pico de gallo, guacamole
  Sour cream.

Procedure:

1. In a bowl, combine the oil (2 Tbsp), lime juice, seasonings, and flavorings, and add the chicken to coat. Refrigerate for 1-2 hrs.
2. In a heavy skillet, sauté the onions and peppers until crisp-tender; do not let them get soft. Remove and cover with aluminum foil.
3. Drain the Chicken, discard the marinade, and in the same skillet, sauté the chicken over medium-high heat until no longer pink, 6 minutes. Add the onion-pepper mixture to warm up.
4. *Serve on the Chickpeas Taco Tortillas. Inspired by* Chickpea Flour Taco Tortillas *inspired by*

Nutrition: Total Fat 16.8g. Saturated Fat 3.2g. Total Carbs 13.8g. Fiber 1.7g. Net Carbs 12.1g. Calories 282 kcal.

Ginger Cashew Chicken Salad

Ingredients for eight servings:

For Chicken marinade

• Protein	Chicken breasts, six oz each #4
• Liquid	Cider vinegar ½ cup
	Molasses 1 Tbs.
	Stevia 3 Tbsp
	Water 1/3 cup
• Fat	Canola oil 1/3 cup
• Seasoning, Flavoring	Ginger root 2 Tbsp
	Soy sauce, low sodium 2 tsp
	Salt 1 tsp
	Ají Amarillo ground ¼ tsp

For the Salad:

- Baby Spinach 8 oz, about 10 cups.
- Mandarin oranges canned drained one can of 11 oz
- Red Cabbage shredded 1 cup.
- Carrots medium shredded two
- Green onion, thinly sliced, three stalks.
- Cashews salted toasted ¾ cup.
- Sesame seeds toasted 2 Tbsp
- Black Bean spaghetti 4 oz

Procedure:

1. In a small bowl, whisk the seven ingredients for the marinade until blended. Pour ¾ cups into a shallow dish or a sealable plastic bag, add the chicken, and turn over to coat. Cover and refrigerate for 3 hours or more. Refrigerate the remaining marinade as well.
2. Cook Black bean spaghetti in boiling water with a small quantity of salt and oil, following the package's instructions, for 4-5 minutes.

3. Preheat the broiler. Drain the chicken, discarding the marinade in the dish. Place the chicken in a baking pan of appropriate size. Broil the chicken at 4-6 inches from the heat source on both sides, 4-6 minutes on each side. The internal temperature should be 165°F. Cut the chicken into strips.

4. Place spinach on a serving platter. Top with chicken, oranges, cabbage, carrots, and green onions. Stir the reserved molasses mixture, drizzle over the salad, and serve.

Nutrition: Total Fat 10g. Saturated Fat 1.3g. Total Carbs 5g. Fiber 0g. Net Carbs 5g. Calories 380 kcal.

Roasted Chicken with Mustard Port Sauce inspired by **(Puck, 2022)**

Ingredients for four servings:

Chicken

- 2 1/2 boneless chickens' thighs
- salt and pepper.
- 3 tbsp olive oil
- two garlic cloves
- one sprig of thyme
- 1/4 cup port wine
- 1/2 cup veal demi-glace
- 1 tsp whole-grain mustard
- 1 tsp Dijon mustard
- 1 tsp of Ají amarillo paste
- water

Salad

- 4 cups mixed greens of your preference.
- 1 tbsp broccolini flowers
- 1/4 cup parsley leaves
- 2 tbsp lemon juice

- 2 tbsp olive oil
- salt and pepper

Procedure:

1. Preheat the oven to 500°F and season chicken with salt and pepper on both sides.
2. Heat a large sauté pan on medium-high heat and coat it with olive oil or nonstick cooking oil spray. When the oil is hot, put the chicken skin side down and cook for 3–4 minutes.
3. When the skin turns golden brown, put the chicken in the oven for 8–12 minutes, depending on its size. When the internal temperature is 165°F, pull the chicken out of the oven.
4. Return to the stovetop and flip over in the pan. Add two garlic cloves and a sprig of thyme to your pan. Baste the chicken with the oil in the pan until the skin is golden brown and the internal temperature reads 165°F.
5. Remove the chicken from the pan and let it rest on a baking rack. Remove the thyme and garlic clove. Now, make your sauce.
6. Place the pan you used for the chicken on medium heat. Deglaze the pan with port wine. Let the alcohol cook out, then add in the veal demi-glace. Whisk the juices together. Reduce for roughly 1 minute. Turn off the heat. Whisk in the whole grain and Dijon mustard. Taste the sauce. Season with salt and pepper if needed.
7. To prepare your salad, combine the mixed greens, broccolini flowers, and parsley leaves in a medium bowl. Drizzle the greens with lemon juice and olive oil. Lightly toss the salad. Season with salt and pepper. Taste.

Nutrition: Total fat 33.8g. Saturated Fat 8.1g. Total Carbs 6.6g. Fiber 1g. Net Carbs 5.6g. Calories 474 kcal.

Alternate Side Dish:

Stir-fried Konjac Fettuccini (may be used as a side dish with any of the entrees).

The Konjac fettuccini is sold under different names; the fettuccini shape works better than the spaghetti shape and does not tangle as much. It has no net carbohydrates, no gluten, and only 4.5 calories per serving. The best and easiest way to prepare them is by stir-frying,

Ingredients for two servings:

- Konjac fettuccini pack 9.5 oz (contains 0 net carbs)
- Scallions (green onions) 4 stems cut small white and light green.
- Frozen green peas 4 Tbsp
- Corn kernels boiled.
- Shallots 1 small, cubed small.
- Neutral favor vegetable oil like avocado or grape seed oil 1 Tbsp
- Ponzu sauce 2 Tbsp

Procedure:

1. Wash the fettuccini in cold tap water in a colander. Allow to dry up in a ventilated area.
2. When the fettuccini is dry, stir fry the shallots for 3-4 minutes; add the scallions, peas, and corn, and warm them up.
3. When warm, add the dry fettuccini and stir fry until a little golden-brown color appears; turn the heat off and add the Ponzu sauce.
4. Serve immediately.
5. If you skip the corn and peas, the carb count drops significantly and can be used with other entre.

Nutrition: Total fat 5g Saturated fat0.4g Total Carbs 16g Fiber 6g Protein 3g Calories 108

Chicken Pan Roasted with Lentils and Cauliflower Rice

Ingredients for four servings:

- Proteins   Chicken Breasts halves 4oz each.
- Carb   Lentils cooked 2 cups.
  Corn kernels frozen ½ cup.
  Salsa or pico de gallo 1 cup
  Cauliflower rice one head.
- Fats   Oil Canola 2 tsp
- Seasoning   Sea Salt ¼ tsp or to taste.
  Pepper Black 1 tsp
- Flavoring agents   Ají Amarillo powder 1 tsp
  Cumin ground 1 tsp
  Cilantro leaves minced 2 tbsp

Procedure:

1. Mix the seasonings and flavorings in a small bowl and sprinkle the mixture over the chicken on both sides. Preheat a large, nonstick skillet, add oil at medium heat, and brown the chicken on both sides.
2. Add the cooked lentils, the corn, and the salsa to the skillet. Cover and cook covered for an internal temperature of 165°F, on average, 10-15 minutes, depending on the size of the chicken breasts.
3. Serve with sautéed cauliflower rice and sprinkle with cilantro.

Nutrition: Total Fat 3.1g. Saturated fat 0.1g. Total Carbs 16.1g. Fiber 5.7g. Net Carbs 10.4g. Calories 216 kcal.

Chicken Tacos with Avocado and Pico de Gallo

Ingredients for four servings:

- Protein   Chicken Breasts, boneless, skinless, cut into stri
- Carbohydrates   Stevia
       Corn kernels 1 cup fresh or frozen
       Eight tortillas inspired by *Chickpea Flour Taco Tortillas*
       inspired by
- Fat   Avocado medium cubed
- Aromatics   Red onion cubed small ½ cup.
       Garlic 3 cloves pressed.
       Tomatoes cherry quartered 1 cup.
- Liquid   Water 1/3 cup.
       Lime juice of ½ lime.
- Seasoning   Sea Salt ½ tsp or to taste.
- Flavoring agents   Ají Amarillo powder 1 tsp
       Oregano 1 tsp
       Cumin 1 tsp
       Paprika smoked 1 tsp.

Procedure:

1. Add water, stevia, seasoning, and flavorings in a large nonstick skillet with cooking spray over medium heat to brown the chicken strips. Cook until chicken is not pink, stirring occasionally, about 4-5 minutes.
2. Meanwhile, in a bowl, mix avocado, corn, tomatoes, and lime juice.
3. Serve over the top of chickpea flour tortillas with salsa. *Chickpea Flour Taco Tortillas*
   inspired by

Nutrition: Total fat 15.5g. Saturated fat 2.6g. Total Carbs 19.4g. Fiber 6.7g. Net Carbs 12.7g. Calories 319 kcal.

Noodles with Peanut Thai Sauce

Ingredients for six servings:

- Protein   Ground chicken meat lean 1 lb.
- Carbohydrates   Pasta Zero Shirataki noodles, three packs.
  Carrots Julienned 1 ½ cup.
  Red Bell Pepper chopped one medium.
  Peanuts unsalted chopped 1 cup.
- Fats   Peanut butter creamy ¼ cup
  Cooking-spray canola or olive oils.
- Aromatics   Green onions chopped, four stalks.
  Garlic 2 cloves pressed.
- Flavoring   Soy sauce reduced sodium ¼ cup.
  Chicken broth, reduced-sodium ½ cup.
- Liquids   Lime Juice fresh ½ cup

Procedure:

1. In a small bowl, mix the peanut butter, the liquids, the flavorings, and the ají amarillo, whisking until blended.
2. Sauté, with cooking spray, the shirataki noodles after rinsing them in cold water and drying them until they appear slightly toasted.
3. In a large skillet with cooking spray, cook carrots, chicken, bell peppers, and garlic over medium heat until the chicken is no longer pink, about 5-6 minutes.
4. Mix peanut butter mix and chopped peanuts, stir this mixture in the skillets, and bring to a boil. Reduce heat to simmering and simmer until sauce has thickened (3-5 minutes).
5. Serve with Shirataki spaghetti and top with green onions.

Nutrition: Total Fat 18.7g. Saturated fat 3g. Total Carbs 16.8g. Fiber 5.4g. Net Carbs 11.4g. Calories 336 kcal.

Chicken Spiced Tortilla Pizza

Ingredients for four servings:

- Protein — Chicken Breasts cut in slices ¾ lb.
  Greek Yogurt plain 1 cup divided.
- Carbohydrates — **Error! Reference source not found.** Or carb
  counter® tortillas (commercially available)
- Fats — Feta Cheese crumbled 2/3 cup.
- Aromatics — Tomato concasse chopped 1/3 cup.
- Flavoring — Fresh cilantro leaves chopped 2 Tbsp+ ½ cup
  Coriander seeds ground ½ tsp.
  Cumin ground ½ tsp
  Ginger fresh grated ½ tsp
  Turmeric ground ½ tsp.
  Paprika sweet ½ tsp
  Ají Amarillo ground ½ tsp

Procedure:

For sauce

1. Mix ½ cup of yogurt with 2 Tbs. of cilantro leaves.
2. Mix the Flavors and ½ cups of yogurt in a large bowl. Stir in the chicken to coat.
3. Place chicken in an oiled grill rack over medium heat; grill covered until no longer pink, about 2-3 minutes per side.
4. Warm the chickpea tortillas.
5. Spread the sauce over the tortillas, top with chicken, cheese, and tomatoes, and sprinkle the remaining cilantro leaves.

Nutrition: Total Fat 5.6g. Saturated fat 2g. Total Carbs 9.7g. Fiber 0.3g. Net Carbs 9.4g. Calories 278 Kcal.

Pan Roasted Chicken Thighs and Vegetables

Ingredients for six servings:

- Protein — Chicken thighs bone in skin in 6 thighs
- Carbohydrates — Parsnips 6, scrubbed and cut into ½-inch pieces.
- Fat — Olive oil light 2 Tbsp
- Aromatics — Onion red large sliced thick one onion
  Garlic cloves pressed three cloves.
- Leafy Vegetables — Baby spinach 6 oz
- Seasoning — Sea Salt 1 ¼ tsp divided.
  Black Pepper ¾ tsp divided.
- Flavoring — Rosemary dried crushed 1 tsp divided.
  Pimenton ½ tsp

Procedure:

1. Preheat oven to 425°F.
2. Combine parsnip, onion, oil, garlic, ¾ tsp salt, and 1/2 tsp pepper in a large bowl. Toss to coat. Transfer to a baking dish 15x10x1 inch, coated with cooking spray.
3. In a large skillet, sauté the chicken thighs until the skin turns golden. Flip over to the other side to reach the same point of doneness.
4. In a small bowl, mix the remaining salt and pepper, rosemary, and pimentón (smoked paprika). Sprinkle this mixture over the chicken and place over the vegetables in the baking dish.
5. Roast in the oven at 425F until the internal temperature of the chicken is 165-170°F.
6. Transfer the Chicken to a serving platter, cover with aluminum foil, and bake the vegetables for another few minutes until the vegetables are tender and the spinach is wilted.
7. Place vegetables on the serving platter and serve.

Nutrition: Total Fat 17.6g. Sat. fat 3.4g. Total Carbs 14.4g. Fiber 4.4g. Net Carbs 10g. Calories 293 Kcal

Fish Recipes

Baked Corvina with Lemon Pepper Crust

Ingredients for two servings:

- Protein   Corvina fillets 8 oz two.
- Fats   Butter 4 tsp
- Seasoning   Lemon Pepper ¼ tsp
                        Sea Salt to taste
- Flavorings   Garlic ½ tsp of powder or one clove pressed.
                        1/8 tsp of pimentón (smoked paprika)
- Liquid   Lemon juice of 1 lemon (2 Tbsp)

Procedure:

1. Preheat oven to 350°F
2. Dry up Fish fillets. Place them in a baking dish bottom sprayed with cooking spray.
3. Pour lemon juice over fillets.
4. Mix seasonings and flavorings in a small bowl and sprinkle evenly over the fish.
5. Place tabs of butter over the fish and bake uncovered to an internal temperature of 135-140°F; the fish meat will be white and flake easily with a fork.

Nutrition: Total Fat 10g. Saturated fat 6g. Carbohydrates 1g. Calories 186kcal.

Quick Braised Fish

Ingredients for four servings:

For the sauce

- Aromatics   Onion sweet one small cubed
  Garlic 2 cloves pressed.
  Ginger 1 cm diced or grated.
- Protein   Fish white meat thick 16 oz (grouper, cod, corvina, etc.)
- Fat   neutral oil of preference (canola or light olive oil)
- Seasoning   Sea Salt and Black pepper to taste
- Flavorings   These will vary depending on the type of sauce you wish to Make. I will give the ingredients at the end of the recipe.

For the fish   Filets of Grouper, cod, or corvina as examples, 4oz each

Procedure:

1. Make the sauce with mild olive oil and the aromatics (onions, garlic, and tomatoes if desired). At this point, you may add other vegetables depending on the sauce you are preparing.
2. Nestle the fish in the sauce and cover it with the vegetables. Put the skillet in the oven and bake at 350°F until an internal temperature of 135-140°F.
3. When the fish is done, remove it and finish the sauce on the top burner at medium-low temperature to thicken, adding herbs and vinegar.

Nutrition: Total Fat 5g. Saturated fat 0.4g Total Carbs 14g Fiber 4g Net Carbs 10g Protein 3g

For different sauces:

- **Puttanesca:** add Ají Amarillo ¼ tsp, tomato paste 1 Tbsp, 14oz Can of tomatoes Marzano or tomato concasse, Basil sprigs, a pinch of stevia, black olives of Botija (Alfonso olives, found in most Latin markets), two tsp of Cappers drained. Nutrition: Fat 1.4g Saturated 0g. Total Carbs 3.7g Fiber 0g

- **Red wine sauce: Add tomato concasse or canned tomatoes three medium, tomato paste 1 Tbsp, red wine ½ cup, carrots, parsnips, mushrooms, chicken broth or beef broth, Basil, and ají amarillo paste 1 tsp Nutrition: Fat 0.3 g Saturated 0g Total Carb 6.3 g** Fiber 1.3g Net Carbs 5 g.
- **Clam sauce:** baby clams 12, clams' juice, white wine ½ cup, ají amarillo ½ tsp oregano, butter unsalted 2 Tbsp, lemon zest two tsp, Italian parsley 2 Tbsp chopped. Nutrition: Total Fat 3.7 g Saturated fat 2.2g Total Carbs 1.5g Fiber 0 g Protein 3.7 g. Calories 75

It may accompany a very low—carb pasta like Zero Pasta®, Healthy noodles®, or SKINNY® with the chosen sauce. Zero Pasta contains 2g of total carbs, all fiber, and zero net carbs.

Cod Soy Sauce Braised

Ingredients for four servings:

- Protein   Cod fillets four of 4 oz each
- Carbs   2 tsp Stevia
- Fat   Sesame oil a drizzle
- Liquid   Fish stock 1 ½ cup
  Mirin 3 Tbsp
  Soy Sauce ¼ cup
- Flavorings   Ají Amarillo
  Habanero chili
  Ginger fresh grated 1 tsp

Procedure:

1. Mix all the ingredients tents except the fish in a small bowl.
2. Brown the surfaces of the fish in a large skillet coated with cooking spray. Remove them from the skillet, replace them with the mixture of the liquids and flavorings, and cook on medium

heat until they begin bubbling. Lower the heat to simmer, place the fish in, and cook to an internal temperature of 135-140°F, flipping them 2-3 minutes after placing them in.

3. Serve over cauliflower fried rice and sprinkle with chopped green onions and braising liquid.

You can replace the soy sauce with any fruit puree you prefer; passion fruit pulp, tamarillo, and mango are my favorites.

Nutrition: Total fat 0.9 g. Sat. Fat 0.3g. Total Carbs 9.8g. Fiber 1.7g. Net Carbs 8.1g. Calories 130 kcal.

Salmon Fillet Roasted

Ingredients for four servings:

• Protein	Salmon fillet with skin 1 lb.
• Fat	Parmesan cheese grated 4 ½ tsp Cooking spray
• Liquid	Lemon juice fresh 2 Tbsp Red wine vinegar 2 Tbsp Soy sauce 1 tsp
• Aromatics	Garlic 2 cloves pressed.
• Flavorings	Grated lemon zest 2 tsp Basil dried 1 ½ tsp. Lemon wedges, four slices
• Seasoning	Black Pepper, a dash

Procedure:

1. Preheat the oven to 350°F.
2. Place the fish skin down in a glass baking pan. Combine the liquids and flavorings in a bowl and pour over the fish. Sprinkle with pepper and parmesan cheese.
3. Bake the fish's internal temperature for 135-140°F for about 15-20 minutes; start checking the temperature at 10 minutes. The time will vary according to the thickness of the fillets. The fish should flake easily when done.
4. Serve with lemon wedges, asparagus, carrots, or noncarb noodles.

Nutrition: Total fat 11g. Sat. Fat 2 g. Total Carb 0g Calories 193 Kcal. Need to add nutrients of side dish used.

Baked Crusted Salmon.

Ingredients for four servings:

- Protein   Salmon fillet skin on 1 ½ lb. center cut.
- Carbohydrates   Stevia 2 Tbsp
  Panko breadcrumbs ¼ cup.
- Fats   Butter unsalted 2 Tbsp
- Aromatics   Garlic clove 1 pressed
- Seasoning   Sea Salt 1 tsp and Pepper ½ tsp
- Flavorings   Paprika sweet ½ tsp
  Ají Amarillo paste 1 tsp
  Parsley leaves chopped ½ cup.
  Dijon mustard 1 Tbsp

Procedure:

1. Preheat the oven to 425°F. Line a baking sheet with aluminum foil. In a small bowl, mix the stevia, aromatics, seasonings, and flavorings. In another bowl, mix the panko crumbs, butter, parsley, ¼ tsp of kosher salt, and a few grinds of black pepper.
2. Place the salmon, skin side down, on the prep baking sheet, spread the surface of the fish with the Dijon mustard, press the stevia mixture over the salmon top, then top with the breadcrumb mixture.
3. Crimp the foil borders to create a border around the fish and collect the juices. Bake until the Panko is golden brown, the salmon is firm and easily flakes, and the internal temperature of the fish is 135-140°F, about 15 to 18 minutes.
4. Serve accompanied by no-carb noodles, cauliflower fried rice, or vegetables of your choice.

Nutrition: Total Fat 18.6 Sat. Fat 5.7g. Total Carbs 9.3g. Fiber 0.3g. Net Carbs 9g. Calories 379 kcal.

Fried rice: fat 4. .7g. saturated fat 0.9g. Carbs 9.1g. Fiber 2.7g. Net 6.4g

Noodles sautéed in cooking spray provide 20 calories, 0 g of fat, 5 g of total carbohydrates, 3 g of Fiber, and 2 g of net carbohydrates.

Fish Tacos

Ingredients for four servings:

- Protein   Mahi-Mahi or cod filets cut into strips 1 lb. Egg large 1
- Carbohydrates   Four tortillas *Chickpea Flour Taco Tortillas inspired by* WASA Crisp Bread, 2
- Fat   ½ cup mayonnaise
- Liquid   skim milk 2 tsp
         Lime juice 1 Tbsp
         Water 1 tsp

Toppings:

- Coleslaw-mix 1 cup
- Tomatoes 2-medium chopped
- Cheese Mexican mix shredded 4 Tbsp
- Cilantro leaves minced 1 Tbsp

Procedure:

1. mix mayonnaise, milk, and lime juice for the sauce and refrigerate.
2. Mix egg and water for an egg wash. Crumble the Wasa® crispy bread.
3. Dip the fish stripes into the egg wash and then into crumbles; pat to adhere.
4. Place a non-stick skillet over medium heat, cover the bottom with cooking spray, add the fish, and cook until golden brown and flakes quickly.
5. Serve in tortillas with toppings and sauce.

Nutrition: Total Fat 10g. Sat. Fat 5g. Total Carbs 12g. Fiber 2g. Net Carbs 10g. Calories

Shellfish Recipes

Mussels in Red Curry

Ingredients for four servings:

•	Protein	Black Mussels scrubbed, debearded 2 lb.
•	Fat	Butter unsalted 2 Tbsp
		Coconut Milk, one 14 oz can
•	Aromatics	Shallots chopped ¼ cup
		Garlic 2 cloves pressed.
•	Flavorings	Madras curry powder 2 Tbsp
		Bay leaves 2
		Parsley leaves Chopped ¼ cup.
•	Liquid	White wine 1 ½ cups
		Lemon Juice 3 Tbsp

Procedure:

1. Melt the butter in a large saucepan over medium heat, then add the shallots and curry powder. Stir until fragrant.
2. Add coconut milk, wine, and bay leaves. Simmer for several (8-10) minutes to allow the flavors to meld.
3. Add the mussels, increase the heat, cover, and simmer until the mussels are open. Remove the mussels into four bowls. Continue to boil the sauce to thicken, stirring, about 2 minutes.
4. Season with salt and pepper, discard the bay leaves, spoon the sauce over the mussels, and sprinkle with parsley or cilantro.

Nutrition: Total fat 5.8g. Sat. fat 3.3g. Total Carbs 5 g. Fiber 0.1g. Net carbs 4.9g. Calories 141 kcal.

Scallops in Parmesan Sauce

Ingredients for four servings:

- Protein   Twelve bay scallops or four sea scallops cut in halves.
- Fats   Unsalted butter 1 Tbsp
  Parmesan cheese four Tbsp
- Flavorings   Lime juice of 2 limes
  Worcestershire sauce 24 drops (1/4 tsp)

Procedure:

1. Use small dishes or small-size ramequins like the ones used for olive oil. Best, scallops' shells.
2. Place the scallops after drying them with paper towels.
3. Squirt lime juice in them.
4. Put three drops of Worcestershire sauce in each.
5. Place a thin slice of butter on top of the scallops.
6. Cover with Shredded Parmesan Cheese
7. Broil on high for 3 minutes or until the surface is golden brown.

Nutrition: Total fat 14.5g. Sat. fat 9.2g. Total carbs: 9g. Fiber 1.9g. Net carbs 7.1g. Calories 209 kcal.

Parihuela Nikei

Ingredients for four servings:

- Protein   Crab meat 8 oz
  Mussels cleaned debearded 12.
  Four squid (7 oz each) Cleaned and cut into rings.
  Sea Scallops cleaned 12.
  Shrimp large shelled and deveined 12.
- Aromatics   Red onions minced in mid-size cubes.
  Garlic 3 cloves pressed.
  Green onions, four spears chopped diagonally.
  Ginger 1 inch peeled and grated.
  Tomatoes Roma, concasse four chopped.
- Fat   Cooking Olive oil 2 Tbsp
- Seasoning   Sea Salt and Black Pepper to taste at the end.
- Flavorings   Ají Panca paste 2 Tbsp
  Waka rehydrated ¼ cup (seaweed)
  Cilantro leaves ½ cup.
  Soy Sauce 1 Tbsp
- Liquid   Lime juice 2 Tbsp
  Fish stock 4 cups
  White wine ¼ cup

Procedure:

1. Heat the oil at mid-heat when shimmering in a large saucepan. Add the onions, garlic, and ginger, and cook until the onions are translucent but not browning.
2. Add the tomato concasse and cook for about 3 minutes, until the tomatoes are soft. Add the ají Panca paste and stir.
3. Add the mussels and cook, stirring for a few minutes.
4. Add the fish stock and the wine, bring to a boil, then add the shrimp, squid, scallops, and fish. Cook until the fish is white and flakes. Remove from the heat.
5. Stir in the wakame, green onions, and crab meat. Garnish with cilantro leaves, drizzle the lemon juice, and serve in bowls. Drizzle a small quantity of virgin olive oil when placing it on the table.

Nutrition: Total fat 12g. Sat. Fat 1.8g. Total Carbs 12.8g. Fiber 1.7g. Net Carbs11.1g. Calories 344kcal.

Scallops Seared with Creamed Corn and Lobster or Lump Crab Meat.

Ingredients for four servings:

- Protein   Sea Scallops large 16
- Carbs   Bell Pepper red and yellow ½ of each julienned
                   Corn sweet yellow ½ cup of kernels
- Aromatics   Garlic 2 cloves pressed.
                   Onion small 2
- Fats   Cooking spray olive oil
                   Heavy cream ½ cup
- Seasoning   Salt and pepper to taste

Procedure:

We will use two pans, one to prepare the sauce and the second to sear the scallops.

For the sauce:

1. Spray a non-stick skillet with cooking spray. Heat the skillet and add the onions and bell peppers. Cook until the onions are translucent but not browning. Then, add the sweet corn kernels and the heavy cream. Cook for 2-3 minutes. At this point, the sauce is almost ready. Add the lump crab meat and cook for another 2 minutes. Reserve and keep warm.

2. Heat the second non-stick pan; when hot, spray the bottom with the cooking spray and place the scallops (cleaned and side muscle removed), allowing sufficient space between them so they will sear and not steam. Do not force the timing of flipping them; if they are adherent to the pan, they are not ready to flip. Check the bottom of the scallops; they should be golden brown. Flip them and repeat the process. Each side will take 2-3 minutes. Alternate the sites in the skillet to use the hottest sites when you flip them.

3. Plate creamed corn at the bottom and scallops on top. Decorate the plate borders with balsamic vinegar reduction. You may top the scallops with julienned fried sweet potatoes.

Nutrition: Total fat6.6g. Sat. fat 3.6g. Total Carbs 21.9g. Fiber 3.3g. Net carbs 18.6g. Calories 153kcal.

Seared Scallops on Cauliflower Puree

Ingredients for four servings:

For the Cauliflower puree

- Carbohydrates   Cauliflower rice 4 cups
  Stevia 1 tsp
- Fat   Cream, Heavy 1 cup
- Aromatic   Garlic 2 cloves pressed
- Seasoning   Sea Salt 1 tsp
  White pepper ¼ tsp
- Liquid   Water 1 quart.

For the dressing

- Carbohydrates   Raisins Golden
  Stevia one pinch
- Fat   Butter, unsalted ½ lb.
  Almonds, toasted, sliced ¼ cup.
- Aromatics   ¼ red onion cubed small
- Seasoning   Sea Salt one pinch
- Flavorings   Capers, minced one tsp.
- Liquid   Red Vinegar 1/4 cup.

For searing the scallops

- Fat   Neutral flavor oil 3 Tbsp
- Protein   Sea Scallops large eight, side muscle removed, dry

Procedure:

Make the puree.

1. Add 1 quart of water, garlic, and salt to a medium sauce pot and heat to a simmer. Then add the cauliflower rice and simmer for ½ hours. Strain well.
2. Place in a blender and puree, slowly adding the cream, until smooth. Season with salt, pepper, and stevia.

Make the dressing.

1. Heat a medium-heavy skillet. The butter will melt, foam, and sizzle at medium heat. When it stops foaming, turn the heat low, and the butter will begin to brown. If it does brown, quickly remove it from the heat momentarily, then back on in low heat until you get the desired color. Add the other ingredients and whisk.

Sear the scallops.

1- Heat a heavy, non-stick skillet. Add the oil and heat at medium heat until the oil shimmers. Then, add the scallops, leaving enough space between them to prevent steaming. Cook each side until the surface is caramelizing and turning golden brown, about 1-2 minutes. Flip them over, preferably when flipping use a different spot in the skillet, where the previous spaces were. Repeat the same process on the second side. You may need to do this in batches.

To serve

-   Place a circular portion of puree; you may use a cooky cutter to shape it well. Place two seared scallops on top of the puree. Drizzle the brown butter vinaigrette over the assembly.

Nutrition: Total Fat 61.6g. Sat. fat 36.3g. Total Carbs 12.3g. Fiber 3.5g. Net Carbs 8.7g. Calories 602 kcal.

Shrimp in Coconut Sauce

Ingredients for four servings:

- Protein   Jumbo raw Shrimp, deveined and shelled 1 ½ lb.
- Fats   Canola oil 5 Tbsp divided (1+2+2).
                 Coconut milk 1 cup
                 Cream cheese softened at room temperature 4-6oz
- Aromatics   Garlic 3 clove pressed.
                 Onion white or yellow ½ coarsely chopped.
                 Bell Pepper red or yellow, seeded and sliced.
                 Tomatoes concasse or canned diced ½ cup
- Seasoning   Sea Salt one tsp
                 Black pepper ground one tsp
- Flavorings   Basil leaves two plus for garnish
                 Cilantro leaves chopped 2Tbsp plus for garnishin
                 Lime Juice of 1 lime
                 Ginger grated one tsp.
                 Paprika, sweet one tsp
                 Ají Amarillo 1 tsp of paste
- Liquid   Chicken or vegetable stock one-third cup

Procedure:

1. In a medium bowl, combine the shrimp, one tablespoon of oil, one clove of garlic, ½ tsp of salt, and ½ tsp of black pepper. Toss and let the shrimp marinate while cooking the aromatics.
2. Heat a heavy, non-stick skillet and add 2 tbsp of oil when hot. When shimmering, add the onions and bell peppers and cook until the onions appear translucent, about 3 minutes.
3. Add the remaining garlic and cook until fragrant, about one minute. Add the tomatoes, concasse or canned, and the cilantro. Cook until tomatoes are soft, about 2 minutes.
4. Transfer the cooked vegetables to a blender and set aside.
5. Add the remaining oil (2 Tbsp) to the same skillet; when the oil is hot and shimmering, cook the shrimp to pink on both sides, about 2 minutes per side. Transfer to a plate and set aside, covered with foil.

6. Add the coconut milk, lime juice, vegetable broth, grated ginger, paprika, and remaining seasonings. Transfer the mixture to a bowl.
7. Add the vegetables and coconut milk mixture to the blender. Blend until the vegetables are ground and the mix is homogeneous.
8. Transfer the contents of the blender to the skillet, bring to a boil, reduce the heat to a simmer, and cook for 5 minutes.
9. Add the cream cheese and mix until melted.
10. Add the cooked shrimp to the skillet and toss to coat. Garnish with the basil leaves and cilantro.
11. Serve over fried cauliflower rice or Pasta zero shirataki noodles.

Nutrition: Total fat 44.7g. Sat. Fat 21.8g. Total Carbs 11.3g. Fiber 2.9g. Net Carbs 8.4g. Calories 469kcal.

Shrimp with Zucchini Noodles

Ingredients for four servings:

• Protein	Shrimp raw 31-40 per lb. one lb.	
• Carbohydrates	Two packets of spiralized zucchini, ten oz each	
• Fats	Butter unsalted 3 Tbsp divided (2 I 1). Olive oil 1 Tbsp	
• Aromatics	Garlic 2 cloves pressed. Shallot one cubed medium.	
• Seasoning	Sea salt ½ tsp. Black Pepper ¼ tsp	
• Flavorings	Cilantro leaves ¼ cup. Lime zest 1 ½ tsp + additional for garnish. Lime Juice 2 Tbsp	
• Liquid	White wine ¼ cup	

Procedure:

1. In a large, heavy, non-stick skillet, melt the 2 Tbsp of butter over medium heat, let it froth away, and then add the shallot. Cook some. Add the garlic and cook until fragrant. Add the lime zest and juice. Continue to cook at medium heat, simmering, not boiling, until the liquid has almost evaporated, 2-3 minutes.

2. Add olive oil and the remaining butter. Stir in the shrimp and, shortly after, the zucchini—season with salt and pepper. Cook until the shrimp turns pink and the zucchini is crisp and tender for about 4 minutes. Sprinkle with parsley and additional lime zest.

Nutrition: Total fat 14g. Sat. Fat 6g. Total Carbs 7 g. Fiber 1g. Net Carbs 6g. Calories 246kcal.

Bibliography

Baier, L. (2019, oct 9). *asweetpeachchef.com.* Retrieved from /chickpea-flour-tortillas/#recipe: https://www.asweetpeachef.com/chickpea-flour-tortillas/#recipe

Canora, M. (2015, Jan 20). */687182/spinach-salad-with-roasted-fennel-and-grapefruit/.* Retrieved from Tasting Table.com: https://www.tastingtable.com/687182/spinach-salad-with-roasted-fennel-and-grapefruit/

Carmellini, A. (2017, Jan 19). */686443/grilled-caesar-cabbage-recipe/.* Retrieved from tastingtable.com: www.tastingtable.com/686443/grilled-caesar-cabbage-recipe/

Chin, K. I. (2019, July). Amigdal NPY Circuits promote the Development of Accelerated Obesity under chronic stress conditions. *Cell Metab.*, 111-128.

Colender, A. (2015, AUG 12). *Tasting Table.* Retrieved from 686998/grilled-radicchio-salad-recipe-yogurt-salad-dressing-grilled-salad-recipe/: https://www.tastingtable.com/686998/grilled-radicchio-salad-recipe-yogurt-salad-dressing-grilled-salad-recipe/

cyafitness.com. (2024). *the-controversy-surrounding-exercises-impact-on-weight-loss-examining-evidence-from-both-perspectives.* Retrieved from cyafitness.com/Articles/: https://www.cyafitness.com/articles/the-controversy-surrounding-exercises-impact-on-weight-loss-examining-evidence-from-both-perspectives

Davis MD, W. (2013). *Wheat Belly Cookbook.* New York, NY: Rodale Books.

Davis, W. M. (2011). *Wheat Belly.* Rodale Books. Retrieved 2023

D'cruz, J. (2023, Jul 24). *nourishing-your-body-and-developing-a-healthy-relationship-with-food/*. Retrieved from earthcycle.io/: https://earthcycle.io/nourishing-your-body-and-developing-a-healthy-relationship-with-food/

Detoximista.com. (n.d.). *cauliflower-pizza-crust/*. Retrieved from https://detoxinista.com/vegan-cauliflower-pizza-crust/: https://detoxinista.com/vegan-cauliflower-pizza-crust/

Fearnley-Whittingstall, H. (1999). *recipes/celeriac-soup*. Retrieved from www.rivercottage.net/: https://www.rivercottage.net/recipes/celeriac-soup

Google Classroom. (2024). *khanacademy.org/science/biology/cellular-respiration*. Retrieved from KhanAcademy.org: https://www.khanacademy.org/science/biology/cellular-respiration--and-fermentation/pyruvate-oxidation-and-the-citric-acid-cycle/a/the-citric-acid-cycle

Hammer, M. (2021, Sept 21). */recipes/86481-cider-braised-chicken-apples-onions-recipe*. Retrieved from https://food52.com: https://food52.com/recipes/86481-cider-braised-chicken-apples-onions-recipe

Hue, L., & Taegtmeyer, H. (2009, Sept 01). *10.1152/aipendo*. doi:10.1152

Keller, T. (2012, Jan 24). *688360/oven-roasted-tomato-recipe-from-chef-thomas-keller/*. Retrieved from //www.tastingtable.com: : https://www.tastingtable.com/688360/oven-roasted-tomato-recipe-from-chef-thomas-keller/

Kevser. (2024, Mar 24). */gluten-free-chickpea-flour-bread-recipe*. Retrieved from //turkishstylecooking.com/: https://turkishstylecooking.com/gluten-free-chickpea-flour-bread-recipe.html

Ko, J. H. (2022 Jun 30; 31(2)). Type 2 Diabetes Remission with Significant Weight Loss: Definition and Evidence-Based Interventions. *J Obes Metab Syndr. 2022* , 123-133. Retrieved from J Obes Metab Syndr. 2022 Jun 30; 31(2): 123–133.

Krampf, R. (2019). *Calories: Measuring the Eneergy*. Retrieved from
the Happy Scientist:
https://thehappyscientist.com/content/calories-measuring-energy

Lagasse, E. (n.d.). */recipes/emeril-lagasse/hot-mayonnaise-glazed-
scallops-3644221*. Retrieved from
https://www.cookingchanneltv.com:
https://www.cookingchanneltv.com/recipes/emeril-lagasse/hot-
mayonnaise-glazed-scallops-3644221

Loh Kim, e. a. (2017). Insulin Controls Food Intake and Energy Balance
via NPY neurons. *Mol Metab.*, 12;6:574-584.

Mucinski, J. (2020, May 15). *doi.org*. Retrieved from doi.org:
https://doi.org/10.1002/lipd.12244

NIH News releases. (2014, 07 08). *www.nih.gov › news-events › news-
releases*. Retrieved from www.nih.gov:
https://www.nih.gov/news-events/news-releases/nih-study-finds-
extreme-obesity-may-shorten-life-expectancy-14-years

Protsiv Myroslava, e. a. (2020, 9: e49555). *PMC/articles*. Retrieved
from www.ncbi.nlm.nih.gov:
https://www.ncbi.nlm.nih.gov/pmc/articles/PMC6946399/

Puck, W. (2022). ROASTED CHICKEN WITH MUSTARD PORT
SAUCE. *MASTER CLASS*.

Revuelta Soba, J. M. (2023). Aquellos tiempos del colesterol. *El Isleño
San Fernando España* , 1-11.

Rider, E. (n.d.). *almond-flour-bread-gluten-free*. Retrieved from
elizabethrider.com: https://elizabethrider.com/almond-flour-
bread-gluten-free

Roberts, C. (2021, Sept 27). *Health/ are-you-addicted-to-sugar-how-to-
beat-sugar-addiction*. Retrieved from www.cnet:
https://www.cnet.com/health/are-you-addicted-to-sugar-how-to-
beat-sugar-addiction/

Robillos, A. (2020, Jul 2). *intermittent-fasting-works/18434/*. Retrieved from tripzilla.ph/: . https://www.tripzilla.ph/intermittent-fasting-works/18434/

Shalaby, Y. M., Aidaros, A. A., & all, e. (2022). Role of ceramides in the molecular Pathogenesis and Potential Therapeutic role in Cardiovascular diseases. *Front Cll Dev. Biol, Sec Cellular Biochemistry*, Vol 9; 2021.

Sivapalan, H. (2022, October 3). *Scolar.google.com.* Retrieved from Adiponectin+levels+(AdipoQ): https://scholar.google.com/scholar?q=Trait:+Adiponectin+Levels+(AdipoQ)&hl=en&as_sdt=0&as_vis=1&oi=scholart

Smith, D. G. (2024, 04 24). */2024/04/24/well/eat/calorie-restriction-fasting-longevity.html*. Retrieved from www.nytimes.com: https://www.nytimes.com/2024/04/24/well/eat/calorie-restriction-fasting-longevity.html

Southern living test Kitchen . (2024, March 11). */recipes/tomato-aspic-recipe*. Retrieved from /www.southernliving.com/: https://www.southernliving.com/recipes/tomato-aspic-recipe

Taste of Home. (20233, september 03). *recipes/beef-burgundy-over-noodles/*. Retrieved from https://www.tasteofhome.com: https://www.tasteofhome.com/recipes/beef-burgundy-over-noodles/

WeightWatchers. (2019, April 22). *food/hormones-appetite-weight*. Retrieved from weightwatchers.com: https://www.weightwatchers.com/au/blog/food/hormones-appetite-weight

Wiss, D. A., Avena, N., & Pedro, R. (2018, 9 18). Sugar Addiction: From Evolution to Revolution. *Front Psychiatry*, p. 545.

Yancy, W. S., Foy, M., & all, e. (2005). A Low-Carbohydrate, Ketogenic diet to treat type 2 diabetes. *Nutr Metab (Lond)*, 2: 34.

INDEX

9 798889 395685 6